Health Psychology in

Health Psychology in Context

Edited by Jo Gilmartin

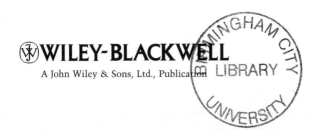

WILEY-BLACKWELL

A John Wiley & Sons, Ltd., Publication

This edition first published 2009 © 2009 John Wiley and Sons Ltd

Wiley-Blackwell is an imprint of John Wiley and Sons, formed by the merger of Wiley's global Scientific, Technical and Medical business with Blackwell Publishing.

Registered office
John Wiley and Sons Ltd, The Atrium, Southern Gate, Chichester, West Sussex, PO19 8SQ, United Kingdom.

Editorial office
John Wiley and Sons Ltd, The Atrium, Southern Gate, Chichester, West Sussex, PO19 8SQ, United Kingdom.

For details of our global editorial offices, for customer services and for information about how to apply for permission to reuse the copyright material in this book please see our website at www.wiley.com/wiley-blackwell.

Library of Congress Cataloging-in-Publication Data

Health psychology in context / edited by Jo Gilmartin.
p. ; cm.
Includes bibliographical references and index.
ISBN 978-0-470-06629-4 (pbk. : alk. paper)
1. Clinical health psychology–Great Britain. I. Gilmartin, Jo.
[DNLM: 1. Chronic Disease–psychology–Great Britain. 2. Psychotherapy–methods–Great Britain.
3. Pain–psychology–Great Britain. 4. Professional-Patient Relations–Great Britain.
WM 420 H4349 2009]
R726.7.H43362 2009
616.001′9–dc22
2008027938

A catalogue record for this book is available from the British Library.
Set in 10.5 on 12.5 pt Sabon by SNP Best-set Typesetter Ltd., Hong Kong.
Printed in Singapore by Fabulous Printers Pte Ltd.
1   2009

Contents

Contributors

Jo Gilmartin is a lecturer in health and psychology at the School of Healthcare, University of Leeds, UK. Her primary research interests focus on day surgery, the risks and benefits of aesthetic surgery and challenges faced by middle managers in the NHS. She is also interested in the consumption and practice of complementary and alternative medicine (CAM) and the evolution and effectiveness of energy psychology interventions.

Joan Maclean is a senior healthcare lecturer at the School of Healthcare, University of Leeds, UK. She teaches health-related psychology and research methods to students from a range of health professions, and her research interests are psychological aspects of illness and high technology care.

Pauline Phillips is a nursing lecturer teaching psychology, communication skills and mental health at the School of Healthcare, University of Leeds, UK. She is also a UKCP registered psychotherapist and has a private practice. Her major research interest is associated with the use of simulated patients in the teaching of communication and counselling skills.

Jenny Waite-Jones is a lecturer in psychology at the School of Healthcare, University of Leeds, UK. Her primary research interests lie within health, and developmental and lifespan psychology. She is particularly interested in the influence of attachment, especially within families, and crossing boundaries between psychology and sociology, as she firmly believes that an individual cannot be understood independently of the social context in which they exist.

Preface

This exciting new book offers a comprehensive in-depth review of theory and research. An attempt is made to offer inspirational content and integrate innovative approaches to practice. This is a deeply considered and lucidly argued health psychology in context book which explores important topics and presents new, remarkable evidence. Health psychology is a prominent topic in the media and government policy debates. There is more interest in tackling obesity, managing acute and long-term conditions, exploring media representations of body image ideals and promoting mental health. In the United Kingdom public health policy is hugely concerned with tackling unhealthy lifestyles and improving health and well-being.

Each chapter offers an up-to-date review, an innovation or empirical data on discrete topics of current relevance and interest in the UK and beyond. The themes are wide ranging and include acute and critical illness, long-term illness, pain psychology, the pressure and impact of the global beauty culture, body image challenges, communication and mental health, family function and health, and challenges faced by health professionals.

This book will be of interest to researchers, educators, health professionals, students in health psychology. It facilitates innovative insights and the updating of professional skills and knowledge in the domain of health psychology. It is a book which offers acts of creation as a way forward for those striving to give quality care to service users with a wide range of health challenges.

Jo Gilmartin

Acknowledgements

We would like to express gratitude to all those who have given help, advice, feedback, encouragement and support in the writing of this book, especially Beth Knight, Emma Lonie, Natalie Meylan, Jackie Ferguson, Janet Jagger, Ted Killan, Ben Grigor and Jonathan White. My thanks also to Bruce Holliday, who did the photography work, and to Philip Yorke, who recruited gym instructors for the photographs. We also wish to thank Dan Halperin and Will Davis for their interest, enthusiasm and participation in the photographs, taken in the University of Leeds gymnasium.

Abbreviations

ADHD	attention deficit hyperactivity disorder
ARDS	acute respiratory distress syndrome
ASMP	arthritis self management programme
CAM	complementary and alternative medicine
CAT	cognitive analytic therapy
CBT	Cognitive behavioural therapy
CDSM	chronic disorder self management programme
CPAP	continuous positive airway pressure
CPN	community psychiatric nurse
CRF	cortisol releasing factor
DMT	dance movement therapy
EBP	evidence-based practice
ECG	electrocardiogram
ED	eating disorders
EDE	eating disorder examination
EDNOS	eating disorders not otherwise specified
EEG	electroencephalography
EFT	emotional freedom techniques
EMDR	eye movement desensitisation and reprocessing
EPP	Expert Patient Programme
ICU	intensive care unit
JIA	juvenile idiopathic arthritis
MRI	magnetic resonance imaging
NICE	National Institute for Health and Clinical Excellence
NSF	National Service Frameworks
PCT	primary care trusts
PEEP	positive end expiratory pressure
PSHE	personal, social and health education
PTSD	post-traumatic stress disorder
RCT	randomised controlled trial
SRRS	Social Readjustment Rating Scale
TPN	total parenteral nutrition

Chapter 1

Introduction: the rainbow of health psychology

Jo Gilmartin

In this book we want, as far as possible, to take the standpoint of exploring contemporary health psychology, providing a comprehensive and rigorous review of theory and new research. Such knowledge will be built up partly by taking account of developments in the new millennium such as the national strategy for health in the UK, and the modernisation agenda. Our aim is also to help promote a deeper and richer understanding of what is involved in the application of psychological principles, rather than add to the stock of interventions that already exist. It is important that healthcare professionals appreciate theoretical constructs underpinning what it is they are trying to do, and why, as well as what evidence base might enable their clinical work to be more effective. Without this, practitioners tend to rely on routine and procedures, and often use the knowledge they do have in ways that are rigid or lacking in perception. If, however, a deeper form of understanding of health psychology is present, health professionals are set free to be more spontaneous and flexible, using their knowledge and unique abilities in confident and creative ways.

This central topic requires us to engage with government policy and strategies for securing good health for the whole population. Globalisation processes too are having a large impact on people's lives resulting in the rapid exchange of ideas, goods capital, information and technologies, and the general compression of distance and time. The dispersal of technology and new knowledge through trade and investment can help in disease scrutiny, treatment and prevention. Moreover information and communications technologies can facilitate swifter access to scientific discovery and evidenced-based practice, enhance knowledge about human rights and strengthen diaspora communities. Contrasting discourses also point to vicious consequences. These include 'the more rapid adoption of unhealthy "Western" lifestyles', and 'globalising new pandemics of tobacco related diseases, obesity and diabetes' (Green and Labonté 2008: 164). Consequently, health professionals need to draw on a range of psychological interventions to deal with the conflict in cultural values, beliefs and attitudes.

In the United Kingdom public health policy has been placed high on the agenda of health and social care agencies concerned with tackling unhealthy lifestyles and improving health. The Wanless review (Wanless 2002, 2004) birthed the *White Paper Choosing Health: Making Healthy Choices Easier* (DH 2004a). It put forward proposals for action on a range of public health issues, including smoking, obesity, and sexual health. Moreover *Choosing Health* made several recommendations for improving food standards and food labelling and the development of healthy schools. Health psychologists too have forefronted theoretical insights to shed light on understanding individual differences in health behaviour (Rutter and Quinn 2002), and these approaches have been useful in health education initiatives (Wardle and Steptoe 2005). In a similar vein, the use of modern information technologies has enhanced the delivery of personalised behaviour change advice. Wardle and Steptoe (2005) emphasise the advantages of delivering health advice through the computer, and the use of image and sound, opening up the learning climate. Despite eloquent strategies to improve health, the implementation process has failed to put forward a workable strategy to reduce inequalities in health, particularly in relation to social, economic and environmental issues (Lloyd et al. 2007). Socio-economic disparities in health seem to prevail.

Beyond this rather obvious statement, there is the current question of how to understand and manage long-term conditions more effectively and a need to appreciate current initiatives towards seeing patients as partners and promoting self-help strategies within healthcare. User-led self-management programmes have grown over the past twenty years. This process encourages patients to voice their opinions, take an active role in their own care and develop creative coping skills. The White Paper *Saving Lives: Our Healthier Nation* (DH 1999) acknowledged the growing evidence of a dynamic role for patients with chronic disease in the management of their own conditions. Moreover in July 2000 the NHS Plan sharpened this initiative through further expansion of the 'Expert Patients' programmes such as greater patient choice and stronger regulation of professional standards (DH 2001).

A corresponding ethic is also embodied in the prevention of major diseases and empowering people to take more control over their health and well-being through making appropriate lifestyle changes. For instance, obesity is a major public health challenge in the 21st century, which now affects developing and industrialised countries alike. Current healthcare frameworks and policy attempt to provide inspiration and direction for tackling the obesity epidemic (DH 2004b, 2007, 2008). The prominence accorded to Western society's exacting standards of physical appearance, and its discriminatory 'anti-fat' attitudes and behaviours, also has major psychological consequences including body image dissatisfaction, social anxiety and poor self-esteem. In effect, tackling obesity is a complex process, focusing on depth psychology to breakthrough emotional drivers, stigmatisation and improved psychosocial functioning. We ought therefore to bear in mind that, in contributing to body image, the consumption of aesthetic surgery is also a pressing concern in health psychology.

This book is exciting and different. For a start, it does not assume that there is a clear-cut and predefined approach to contemporary health psychology which we need to carefully describe and explain. Rather, the writers take a risk and explore disparate subjects, arriving at a threshold that is central, fascinating and evolving. The book was conceived and produced in the spirit of conceptual creativity with a desire to provide a better understanding of 21st century health psychology; and significantly, to analyse health psychology in transition. More recently, critical attention has turned to energy psychology, and especially its usefulness in treating emotional and physical symptoms including anxiety, addictions and eating disorders, thus holding the potential to revolutionise psychology. Energy psychology methods might seem wacky; nonetheless, attempts will be made to elucidate the detail and intricacy that make up this apparently ever-fascinating field.

About the chapters

Although very much in the present in tone, Chapter 2 draws on psychological factors which may be common to acute/critical illness, and discusses possible responses to specific conditions or situations. It examines the stress of being acutely ill, and that associated with the period of recovery. Acutely ill patients will be subject to highly invasive interventions to support them during critical periods, therefore aspects of critical illness psychology is explored, including classic notions of intensive care unit (ICU) syndrome, but also more recent ideas, such as psychological adjustment following a period of severe illness, and the possibility of post-traumatic stress disorder (PTSD) symptoms following time in intensive care. The concluding section looks at the impact of sophisticated technological devices on psychological well-being.

Chapter 3 includes consideration of long-term illness, with particular emphasis on the importance of adopting a bio-psycho-social approach. The social context of chronic illness is considered in terms of health inequalities and related stressful experiences. Links between stress and chronic illness, evident within psycho-neuroimmunology, are explored and the importance of social support, as well as other useful interventions, discussed. Finally, the extent to which the 'voice of the patient is increasingly being recognised within healthcare through current initiatives within the National Health Service, including the Expert Patient Programme, patient education, patient professional partnerships and other self-help strategies, is appraised.

Chapter 4 condenses the vast amount of literature students might encounter when seeking information about the psychology of pain. How do pain theories link with observed behaviours? What psychological concepts can really help us understand individual responses to pain, and have they been drawn upon in practice? We look at the impact variables such as gender and personality might have on pain response, and the different psychological factors involved in so-called acute and chronic pain states. Finally psychological interventions which may be useful in addition to pharmacology are explored.

In Chapter 5, body image is examined, exploring media representation and the challenging area of appearance-related concerns and the consequences on well-being. In line with media representations, the 'beauty standard' benchmark is considered and its impact on psychological function, attitude and behaviour. In the theoretical spirit, gender and teenager representations are explored too, revealing the anxieties, insecurities and possibilities for transformation tied to the 'beauty aesthetic'. Eating disorder behaviours such as anorexia nervosa and bulimia are investigated and psychological interventions for treating them are offered, including music therapy, art therapy and dance therapy.

Chapter 6 is grounded in the context of women's and men's dissatisfaction with their bodies, exploring the threats and risks of obesity. Psychodynamic explanations of obesity are considered in conjunction with examining how environments, genes and behaviour interact to cause obesity. A variety of psychological interventions and educational strategies, broadly conceived, are brought together here, approaches that are useful in prevention and treatment for children and adults. The weighing-up of evidence involves focusing on the use of physical activity combined with dietary change, exploring emotional states in regard to eating patterns and the effectiveness of cognitive behavioural techniques and bariatric surgery. Body modification with its comforting position of 'self enhancement' is explored briefly drawing on cosmetic surgery, tattoos and piercing. Acquired disfigurements and altered body image as a result of head and neck cancer, facial trauma, and the impact of chemotherapy on hair loss will be examined. Although quite specific, they often contribute to the messy, brutal and distressing psychological frame related to anxiety, low self-esteem and depression. Yet while there is a theoretical bent to despair, attempts are made to increase self-efficacy and encourage social integration. This leads on to more insidious changes, as in the ageing process and its impact on attractiveness and sexuality.

Chapter 7 considers mental health and well-being focusing on what mental health is, how it is developed and how it is threatened. The interaction between mental health and human relationships will be considered from different psychological perspectives and application to healthcare will be considered. Healthcare professionals are regularly confronted with people suffering pain, disease, injury, trauma, loss and grief, experiences associated with poor mental health. It can be challenging and difficult to communicate therapeutically with people experiencing such problems. However, healthcare professionals can be helped to address this often-neglected aspect of their work through knowledge and understanding of theoretical frameworks which illuminate human communication and relationships. Interventions which may be employed in the promotion of mental health in all healthcare settings will be discussed.

The final two chapters focus on the challenges and stressors encountered by health professionals, and the corresponding strain of childhood chronic illness and disability on family function. In this context, challenges faced by both professional and lay carers are examined. Chapter 8 includes a look at family processes and how these are affected by illness or disability. The impact on different family members, including changing family roles and responsibilities over the family life-cycle is explored. Finally, current initiatives and interventions within healthcare which recognise and meet the needs of patients within their family context, as well as specific support strategies to aid family adjustment, are discussed.

Chapter 9 examines the challenges faced by health professionals in attempting to change health beliefs and health behaviour, especially in people troubled by body image dissatisfaction or those plagued by obesity. Innovative interventions including emotional freedom techniques (EFT) are explored, suggesting techniques for changing belief systems. The motives and intentions of the health professional are discussed in the process of helping patients change their predicament drawing on the idea of a 'script' as revealed through the conception of transactional analysis. This chapter moves from concern with 'script' behaviour of health practitioners for emotional well-being, and the consequences of low vibrational frequency. Suggestions are offered concerning ways to climb the emotional scale and focus on deliberate intent. An overview is given of the usefulness of interventions such as evidence-based practice, web-based information and energy psychology including EFT for changing health behaviour.

References

Department of Health (DH) (1999) *Saving Lives: Our Healthier Nation*. London: The Stationery Office.

Department of Health (DH) (2001) *The Expert Patient: A New Approach to Chronic Disease Management for the 21st Century*. London: Department of Health.

Department of Health (DH) (2004a) *Choosing Health: Making Healthy Choices Easier*. London: The Stationery Office.

Department of Health (DH) (2004b) *Initiatives to Promote Healthier Lifestyles*. Accessed 2 July 2007 http://www.dh/gov.uk .

Department of Health (DH) (2007) *Obesity Team/Health Improvement Directorate*. Accessed 20 August 2007 http://nationalobesityforum.org.uk.

Department of Health (DH) (2008) *Healthy Weight, Healthy Lives, a Cross-government Strategy for England*. Accessed 20 February 2008 http://www.dh/gov.uk policy/guidelines.

Green J. and Labonté R. (2008) *Critical Perspective in Public Health*. London: Routledge.

Lloyd C.E., Handsley S., Douglas J., Earle S. and Spurr S. (2007) *Policy and Practice in Promoting Public Health*. London: Open University Press, Sage.

Rutter D. and Quine L. (eds) (2002) *Changing Health Behaviour*. Buckingham: Open University Press.

Wanless D. (2002) *Securing our Future Health: Taking a Long-term View*. London: HMSO.

Wanless D. (2004) *Securing Good Health for the Whole Population*. London: HMSO.

Wardle J. and Steptoe A. (2005) Public health and psychology. *The Psychologist* 18(11): 672–5.

Chapter 2

Acute and critical illness

Joan Maclean

Introduction

This chapter explores the psychological impact on the patient of a period of acute or critical illness. The stress which may be engendered by acute illness and spill over into recovery is discussed. Psychological aspects of intensive or critical care are examined, as is the notion of post-traumatic stress as induced by this experience. The chapter does not include detailed comment on stress as a factor in the development of illness; for helpful discussion of this the reader can access a number of health psychology texts, including Marks et al. (2000) or Weinman et al. (2006).

The patient is an individual with physiological, social and psychological needs, and the onset of acute or critical illness brings about a sudden and marked change to these. We endeavour as health professionals to assist in the meeting of patients' needs, and the scope for psychology in the care of the acutely ill patient is wide. Indeed the National Institute for Health and Clinical Excellence (2007) guidelines on care of the acutely ill patient in hospital recommend specifically that psychological and emotional needs of the patient are included in all formal handovers of care. The ability to anticipate and interpret a patient's requirements, and to detect potential distress, are desirable skills in anyone caring for the acutely ill, and an understanding of the application of psychology to the situation supports and strengthens these skills.

Technology-assisted treatment

Enormous changes in healthcare have taken place during the past two decades. Strong evidence of these changes can be seen in the fields of acute and intensive care, where science and engineering have been harnessed by health professionals in the attempt to support and prolong life. Advanced technology has led to the admission of increasingly sicker patients to hospital wards and units, and, consequently, to patients surviving any number of perilous events in the course of their disease. Without doubt the experience of the acutely ill patient can be a forbidding one. Despite the clear intention on the part of healthcare staff to provide help and support, the hospital can be a frightening place, in particular perhaps the intensive or high dependency unit. Even healthcare professionals inured to hospital sights and sounds, but new to intensive care, may remark on the alien and intimidating nature of the environment. What then for the patient on the receiving end? This rapid evolution of technology-assisted treatment has meant that high technology environments appear throughout hospitals, and are familiar areas to staff, yet they may remain a potentially upsetting and strange experience for both patients and their families.

Stress and acute illness

Perspectives on stress have evolved through various stages, from the response and stimulus based approaches, through to the transactional or cognitive-phenomenological approaches in contemporary psychology. There are aspects of each approach which can be useful to health professionals, and readers will find stress discussed in a biological context in Chapter 3. A transactional approach to stress – as, for example, the model posited by Richard Lazarus and Susan Folkman (Lazarus 1966, 1981; Lazarus and Folkman 1984), combines aspects of the response-based and stimulus-based models, and in particular introduces the notion of mediators. It sees stress in terms of interaction between person and environment. Here subjectivity becomes important; the potentially stressful event is cognitively appraised by the individual with factors such as experience, personality, available social support and relative importance entering the equation. This appraisal process results in perceived demand set against perceived coping ability, and where the former outweighs the latter stress will be experienced. Reversal of the equation means stress will be minimal or absent.

   It can be seen then that the all-important factor in the transactional approach to stress is individual perception of circumstances – an aspect not fully considered by a wholly response-based or stimulus-based approach. For example, the response-based notion of generalised adaptation as proposed by Selye in 1956 made little allowance for any individual elements, such as cognitive variables, which might temper and vary stress response in individuals. Though psychological stress may be mapped onto the general adaptation syndrome, psychosocial elements cannot be fully incorporated. The generalised adaptation syndrome shows *how* we respond to psychological stress, but perhaps not *why*. Nevertheless it remains a useful model to illustrate a number of physically stressful experiences. Meanwhile the stimulus-based approach to stress exemplified by such measures as the Social Readjustment Rating Scale (SRRS or Life Events scale: Holmes and Rahe 1967) tends to offer an objective view of stress, and therefore leaves gaps in the subjective areas of individual or personal experience.

Stress appraisal

The 'stress and coping' model proposed by Lazarus suggests a primary appraisal of the situation, where events are classified as 'irrelevant', 'relevant and positive', or 'relevant and negative' – in other words threat to the individual is calculated and 'relational meaning' is assessed (Lazarus 1999). 'Relevant and negative' constitutes a stressful appraisal. Secondary appraisal of the event involves evaluation of options and capacity for coping with presumed threat. In essence there is a dynamic relationship between demands and resources which may be altered at any time as a result of some significant event. This appraisal system furnishes an explanation for individual differences in experience of stress. Learning, memories, personalities, perceptions of control and social support, and of the significance of events, vary tremendously and alter overall meaning for each person. The lone parent accompanying a child to hospital during a first, unheralded asthma attack may experience stress on an apparently greater level than the supported parent whose child has suffered and recovered from numerous similar attacks; by the same token, then, illness (which is ranked sixth on the SRRS) will engender different levels of stress for different patients depending on the layers of meaning attached at cognitive appraisal. Is this an exacerbation of a chronic condition – say an infection episode in a patient with airways disease – in which case there may be a degree of previous experience, or is it a new, sudden onset condition like a first myocardial infarction or acute cholecystitis, where the previous experience involved in cognitive appraisal is minimal? Lazarus (1999) uses the term 'relational meaning' to describe this combination of subjective appraisal and personal significance of a situation; it is this which allows the individual to calculate the degree of threat imposed to their wellbeing and may determine in part their outwardly manifest reaction to the situation.

More recent is the development of a cognitive phenomenological perspective to explain stress. This suggests that emotion and cognition are so dependent upon personal experience that their mediating role is best understood using a phenomenologically based approach. Motivation and goal-directedness may influence response (Pervin 1989, Cantor et al. 1991) and also the individual's 'world view' – individual attitudes and beliefs about the world – may impart meaning within the transaction (Scheier and Carver 1987, Janoff-Bulman 1989, Wortman et al. 1992). Janoff-Bulman (1989) has described an 'assumptive world' wherein each of us has a set of schemata which furnishes us with the information by which we function on a daily basis. The cognitive phenomenological perspective proposes then that individual differences in world view might account for varied reactions to stressful experiences, while mental constructs which make up the 'assumptive world' may become vulnerable in extreme stress, such as that experienced by the acute and critically ill. Becoming acutely ill, and undergoing a variety of invasive procedures and treatment options, may result in a distressing unravelling of constructs. Where once the individual – if they considered their health at all on any regular basis – saw themselves as hale and hearty, now they have to face a different world, albeit maybe temporary, in which their health is quite a fragile thing and their wellbeing is threatened.

The intensive care experience

The intensive care unit (ICU) exists within a hospital to provide specialised care for patients requiring respiratory support via mechanical ventilation, and/or treatment of organ failure. Patients admitted to this area will generally need treatment for some life-threatening yet potentially reversible condition; alternatively they may need support pending a definitive diagnosis, or while waiting to undergo surgery or receive an organ transplant. The majority of ICUs in the United Kingdom are staffed by specialised teams comprising intensive care trained medical and nursing staff, plus technical and administrative personnel. There will also be access to physiotherapists, pharmacists, radiographers, dieticians and other health professionals, all with specific experience in the care of the critically ill patient. A senior medical practitioner with specific intensivist training, and a senior nurse, will usually be in overall charge of the unit. Patients may also be under the care of the admitting surgeon or physician and their teams, thus the ICU tends to function with a considerable degree of crossover of care, so that the patient's management will be influenced by a number of people.

Respiratory failure results in hypoxia (lack of oxygen supply to tissues) and very often in retention of carbon dioxide. Oxygen delivered via face mask or nasal cannulae may be administered in an attempt to treat hypoxia, but if respiratory failure cannot be dealt with satisfactorily by oxygen inhalation therapy then mechanical ventilation of the lungs may be required. Here a prescribed composition of gases is blown into the lungs via an endotracheal tube which has been introduced nasally, orally or via tracheostomy, allowing both the delivery of gases and the suction removal of secretions. Variations on this approach to ventilation may be used in order to optimise patient recovery – for example elevation of airway pressure during expiration, either by way of applying positive end expiratory pressure (PEEP) to the ventilator, or by connecting the spontaneously breathing patient to a continuous positive airway pressure (CPAP) system.

Aside from respiratory support, general management of the acutely ill patient involves a range of procedures which collectively contribute to the potentially stressful experience. Circulatory support may require invasive monitoring by way of central venous, radial and pulmonary arterial catheterisation; bladder catheterisation will be necessary to monitor renal function, and if that function becomes grossly impaired then artificial haemofiltration may be required. Maintenance of nutrition might be by enteral feeding via a nasogastric tube; alternatively a dedicated central venous catheter will be inserted to allow total parenteral nutrition (TPN) – infusion of a solution of protein, carbohydrate, fat, electrolytes, vitamins, trace elements and water.

Psychological well-being of the acutely ill

All of these life-supporting measures may be potentially traumatic or stressful enough to impact collectively on the emotions and psychological wellbeing of the acutely ill. The intubated patient, who cannot speak because the endotracheal tube passes through the vocal cords, may be too disorientated or incapacitated to communicate adequately by non-verbal means. Self-ventilating patients, too, may be exhausted, confused, or receiving strong medication, rendering them unable accurately to communicate with people and report pain, discomfort or anxiety. Those admitted electively, for example for surgery, are likely to have received at least some information in advance – although the sensation of waking attached to a ventilator may be a shock even to the best prepared patient. Unplanned admission in the event of acute illness, however, may mean that procedures such as intubation, ventilation, catheterisation and insertion of lines have taken place under emergency conditions and little or no psychological preparation will have been possible.

Pain relief is fundamental to management; pain may arise both from the initial clinical problem as well as from the invasive procedures involved in support and monitoring, requiring the infusion of opiates or their derivatives. The chosen combination of analgesia and sedation will vary according to the clinical picture, unit policy and individual practice. Specific and more detailed discussion of psychological aspects of pain can be found in Chapter 4. While controlling pain, anxiety and distress must also be minimised; management of the critically ill patient will include as an imperative assessment of the apparent level of sedation and comfort. Scoring systems may be used to quantify level of sedation by way of motor activity and response to stimuli.

The need for sedative drugs may vary: some patients by nature of their disease may be minimally conscious, others may be awake but tolerant of the ventilator, and receiving adequate pain relief yet apparently alert. In the ICU context sedation may be aimed both at sleep, and at the relief of anxiety when the patient is awake. Anxiolytic drugs may be given, and in the longer-staying patient who needs to reset a sleep/waking pattern, simple night sedation may be administered.

Control as a mediating variable

Control is an important mediating variable involved in the appraisal of stress, and it is interesting to consider how this might be applied to acute and critical illness situations. The loss of control engendered by stressful situations appears to result in certain stress-related physiological and psychological effects which influence both health and emotional status (Rotter 1966; Stewart and Salt 1981; Fisher 1984); certainly the transactional model places emphasis on perceived control as a determinant of experienced stress. Sudden death in humans, related to unmitigated and uncontrollable stress, has been described in various studies (Engel 1971; Mittelman et al. 1995). Such dramatic outcomes may be relatively rare; nevertheless perceived lack of control over aversive and stressful situations has distressing effects. Animal psychology experiments have generated a number of findings in the field, subject to some controversy. Brady et al. (1958) examined the effects of uncontrollable stress on rhesus monkey pairs subjected to intermittent electric shocks. Both monkeys had access to a pressable bar: the 'executive' could thereby postpone shock while the yoked monkey's efforts had no effect. At post mortem the executive subjects exhibited severe peptic ulceration while the yoked monkeys had sustained a significantly lower amount of physiological damage. These findings were at the time extrapolated to human behaviour, and yet the Brady experiment appears to contradict any notion of a link between loss of control and greater stress – though it emerged on close examination of the methodology that the more nervous or active monkeys had been assigned to executive roles, thus the yoked monkeys were very possibly more placid, introducing the confounding question of temperament and its link with stress.

Predictability – or lack of it – of an aversive event is closely linked to controllability; this aspect was explored by Weiss (1970). Predictability of shock was manipulated among three groups of rats, which received shock randomly, received shock with warning, or were no-shock controls. Here peptic ulceration arose in 100%, 67% and 25% of the groups respectively, accompanied by highest corticosteroid release, core temperature and weight loss in the unpredictably/randomly shocked group. The conclusion here was that predictability could modify response to equal doses of stress, despite the absence of control. The introduction of controllability of shock, by using executive:yoked pairs, resulted in greater ulceration in the yoked rats, the reverse of Brady's findings. Here the element of control appeared to lend a buffering effect (Weiss 1971a).

Stress and learned helplessness

Further aspects of uncontrollable stress have been explored in experimentally induced states of learned helplessness (Seligman et al. 1971) where dogs subjected to unavoidable painful electric shocks in a pre-test situation were unable to learn avoidance behaviour when shocks were administered where escape was possible. The premise is that learned helplessness develops when outcome is not contingent on performance, and this is then generalised to other stressful and aversive situations where avoidance is in fact possible. Learned helplessness has been explored in relation to hospital experience: Raps et al. (1982) felt it could be brought about by hospitalisation, although participants in their study of both inpatients and outpatients, while 'not chronic patients', were not included where treatment plans were less than several months.

Extrapolation of findings from animal psychology is of course questionable, yet effects similar to those noted by researchers like Brady, Weiss and Seligman have been demonstrated in human subjects. The ability to predict stressful events may reduce emotional disturbance, and studies in clinical settings have borne this out (Siegel and Peterson 1980; Taylor 1982). Peterson and Seligman (1984), examining risk factors for depression, argued the importance of perceived control in the onset of depression; if an individual perceives, rightly or wrongly, hopelessness or lack of control in the face of stressful or aversive situations then he or she will learn helplessness.

The acutely ill patient

If change is stressful, and control and predictability are important factors in stress, where can we use these theories and findings in relation to the acutely or critically ill patient? This group of patients may be subjected to all manner of distressing events, all engendering change, many unpredicted, and quite possibly allowing the minimum of perceived control. Occurrences within the high dependency or intensive care unit, coupled with the consequences of acute or critical illness, may generate a great deal of stress for those who survive. Conceptual frameworks which seek to explain stress and post-traumatic stress can offer the healthcare practitioner a great deal of help in understanding the experience of the acutely ill patient, and may enhance the care they offer. As with any stressful life event, some individuals may be able to digest and absorb the experience of acute illness more readily than others.

A great deal of literature is available which centres on the psychological problems inherent in the treatment and management of the critically ill (Kornfeld 1969; Ashworth 1980, 1984, 1990; Simpson-Wilson 1987; Dracup 1988; Dyson 1999; Strahan and Brown 2005); a similarly large body of research exists which focuses on the considerable emotional strain experienced by the relatives or 'significant others' of patients (Molter 1979; Coulter 1989; Wilkinson 1995; Engstrom and Soderberg 2004). The psychological sequelae of a period in intensive care have been considered within a number of studies and from a range of perspectives over the years (Kornfeld 1969; Jones and O'Donnell 1994; Thiagarajan et al. 1994; Jones, Humphris and Griffiths 1998; Schelling et al. 1998; Nickel et al. 2004). A short stay or a relatively minor event might evoke as much, and sometimes more, distress than an extended, full-scale experience of the ICU, bearing out the tenets of the transactional model of stress as outlined above.

Stress experienced in acute illness is multifaceted and may be produced by such factors as pain, fear, social isolation and immobility, helplessness and ineffective communication – all over and above the generalised debilitation associated with the disease or condition itself. A degree of immobility may be an unavoidable feature of highly monitored care involving oxygen or ventilation tubing, nasogastric tubes, urinary catheters, intravenous, intra-arterial and intracranial cannulae, and electrocardiogram (ECG) leads. Indeed the treatments and procedures attendant upon ICU admission, should this be necessary, have been compared to torture by Dyer (1995) in the context of ICU delirium states.

Responses such as depression, anxiety, confusion and delirium may result in part from a mix of sensory overload and sensory deprivation. It has been noted that the psychotic symptoms exhibited by some patients parallel those induced by sleep deprivation and some categories of psychological torture, such as isolation or exposure to white noise (Dyer 1995). Sleep disturbance alone can result in psychological problems on discharge to the ward, with patients reporting restlessness, memory and judgement impairment (Dracup 1988; Topf et al. 1996). Certainly noise and activity within the ICU may have negative effects on sleep for recovering patients, rendering them liable to confusion and weariness. Further, given the importance attached to sleep with regard to restoration of energy and reinforcement of protein synthesis and immune function (Horne 1988; Topf et al. 1996) attention to noise levels and promotion of sleep are clearly important aspects of intensive care.

Psychological impact of intensive care

In 1966 McKegney described what was then referred to as ICU psychosis – a 'madness in ICU', an unfortunate spin-off of medical progress. Such early reports of psychosis emerged from observation of patients undergoing cardio-pulmonary bypass for open heart surgery, in whom a high rate of hallucination, agitation and confusion was documented. Much of this psychological disturbance was related to the disorientating and threatening environment within early cardiothoracic ICUs (Solomon et al. 1957; McKegney 1966). Kornfeld (1969) observed that in many patients symptoms were alleviated on transfer back to the standard hospital ward. This was one of the first studies to make recommendations in relation to psychological disturbance, in particular encouragement of uninterrupted rest or sleep periods, reduction of unnecessary noise and light, particularly at night, and an attempt to orientate patients by way of clocks, calendars and a view through an outside window wherever possible. Some of the neuropsychological consequences of cardiac surgery may have been attributable to the use of cardiopulmonary bypass itself and the attendant risks of reduced cerebral perfusion and microembolism (Abram 1965; Taylor 1982; Mills and Prough 1991), which could explain some of the observations of ICU psychosis in cardiac surgery patients, certainly in earlier reports.

Though some of the bizarre sensory experiences within ICUs have been minimised today – for example twenty-four hour full lighting is viewed with disfavour, and the (controlled) presence of relatives is now generally encouraged – a hyperactive delirium may still occur wherein the conscious patient displays fear, agitation, confusion and disorientation (Hopkinson and Freeman 1988; Dyer 1995; Devlin et al. 2007; Pun and Ely 2007). Hypoactive or 'quiet' delirium, where the patient is passive, with a flat affect – that is, reduction in emotional expression and psychomotor slowing – is equally important yet perhaps harder to recognise. Certainly delirium is a complication, arising during the acute period of illness within the ICU, which has the potential for repercussion in the recovery period.

Even in the absence of exaggerated responses, individuals may still display some adverse reaction to the stress generated by the ICU experience. Patients may be deprived of meaningful sensory input yet simultaneously exposed to a battery of strange, uninterpretable stimuli leading to sensory imbalance. Sensory overload or overstimulation, in general terms, occurs as a result of bombardment by higher than normal levels of stimulation, frequently in more than one modality and often sudden and unpredictable (Goldberger 1986). Potential sensory overload in the ICU could be produced by a range of things – for instance, the repetitive sounds of ventilators, the noise produced by infusion pumps and filtration equipment, alarms on most machinery, and the unfamiliar noise and activity associated with these areas. In the 1970s exposure to noise in excess of 70 decibels was reported (Bently et al. 1977); the recommended limits now are much lower. In addition the stimulation by way of treatment procedures should be considered; these could conceivably feel sudden and unpredicted to the sick patient, despite the best efforts of staff to prepare and inform. Endotracheal suction, insertion or removal of lines, chest X-rays, physiotherapy and general nursing care make up routine and necessary care, and yet they are unfamiliar sensations, which may happen frequently and become potential stressors. In conjunction with this sensory overload, sleep disruption may compound all the other stressful factors impinging on the ICU patient. A proactive approach is adopted now to make every effort to minimise disruption, including noise reduction, attention to rest and sleep patterns, early mobilisation and cognitive stimulation, and screening of patients for confusional states.

Recall after discharge

Recall may also be a feature of the recovery period after intensive care, and may be affected by a number of factors, including the mixture of drugs administered, and altered cerebral perfusion brought about by haemodynamic instability. 'Awareness' versus 'recall' are worth differentiating: Cheng (1996) has defined awareness as a state of awakeness and cognisance, and recall as explicit memory for events. Egerton and Kay (1964) undertook one of the earlier reported studies of recall for events while critically ill, an examination of patients discharged from a respiratory support unit. They found evidence of patient recall for several details of care, including unpleasant memories of endotracheal suction and arterial blood sampling. Hewitt (1970) found that although around 65 patients from a sample of 100 could say how long their stay in ICU had been, more than 70 could not recall major procedures like ventilation or extubation. For those who did demonstrate recall, procedures such as endotracheal suction, and removal or manipulation of drainage tubes were quite vivid and concerning. Interestingly there was little difference in recall between those patients who were mechanically ventilated and those who managed spontaneous respiration.

More recently Holland et al. (1997) studied patients' recollections and satisfaction with care received in the ICU: despite some vivid memories, those patients who reported the least stress from the experience were those who recalled staff demonstrating caring attitudes and an ability to anticipate needs. From the literature, it does seem that a significant proportion of survivors are able to remember particularly stimulating moments of the treatment received in the ICU, and Cheng (1996) suggested that suppression of awareness and recall might help prevent psychological problems following discharge from the unit. Yet the difference between real and mistaken recall is important, and Jones et al. (2001) suggest that memories for genuine events may in fact help to protect against anxiety, and that it may be delusional memories rather than factual memories which are associated with PTSD-related symptoms following discharge from the ICU, as discussed below.

Post-traumatic stress and illness

An associated area of study is the potential for patients who have survived an episode of acute illness, particularly where high-dependency or intensive care has been received, to suffer from symptoms related to post-traumatic stress disorder (PTSD). This is a long-term consequence of an acutely stressful and traumatic experience, and its defining feature is the development of characteristic symptoms after an overwhelming event. These symptoms fall into three main clusters: the first are symptoms associated with intrusive thought and reliving of the trauma, the second with avoidance, where the sufferer tries to minimise exposure to reminders, and the third cluster relates to hyperarousal – that is symptoms such as hypervigilance, increased startle response and insomnia (DSM IV American Psychiatric Association 1994). In addition emotions such as anger, sadness, shame or guilt may be reported (Brewin et al. 1996), often depending on the nature of the traumatic event preceding the syndrome.

Clearly this is an uncomfortable state to endure. Physiological as well as psychological symptoms may be present. Some symptoms can be understood in the context of the stress response, discussed earlier in this chapter, and also in Chapter 3. The symptoms of anxiety and hyperarousal, such as increased muscle tension, heightened alertness, sleep disturbance and hypervigilance, indicate a prolonged state of stress resistance, fuelled by continued outpouring of stress hormones. Lovallo (1997) has remarked that the central nervous system mechanisms which integrate the physiological stress response may be subject to long-term changes in cases of PTSD, as a result of alteration in connections between frontal lobe and limbic system, and in brainstem feedback to the central nervous system.

Like most psychological phenomena, PTSD can be viewed from a number of perspectives. A variety of conceptual models exists to furnish explanations of the specific symptoms. Biological or physiological factors have been suggested, including the impact of raised cortisol releasing factor (CRF) and cortisol levels, and reduced serotonin uptake (Pitman 1997), and the effect on memory storage of excessive noradrenaline release at and around the time of the trauma (Hagh-Shenas et al. 1999).

Keane et al. (1985) have adopted a behavioural approach to assessing and treating PTSD, and explain its development by way of both classical and operant conditioning. The hyperarousal seen in PTSD may be brought about by classical conditioning if, during the illness period, a neutral stimulus has been paired with some extremely painful or unpleasant unconditioned stimulus. The previously neutral stimulus becomes a conditioned stimulus, which may evoke activation of the autonomic nervous system and an adrenaline evoked response. This concept of classical conditioning is explained in some further detail in Chapter 4.

With regard to operant conditioning, traumatic and distressing experiences are inherently aversive, and the majority of us would not wish to repeat them given a choice. Keane suggested that the avoidance behaviour adopted by PTSD sufferers may be explained simply by way of negative reinforcement. That is, repeated avoidance of situations, conversations and the like will prevent the unpleasantness of remembering and reliving events.

Cognitive appraisal models as described earlier (Janoff-Bulman 1985, 1989; Epstein 1990) view PTSD as a result of the disruption of assumptive constructs. Strongly held beliefs in the world, which are summarised by Janoff-Bulman (1985) as our notions that the world is comprehensible and controllable, benevolent in the main, and that each individual is worthy and largely invulnerable, are shattered by the experience of a threatening event. The more devastating the damage to schemata, that is the more incongruent the trauma-related information with pre-existing ideas about life, the more work required to repair and reconstruct. The immense cognitive mismatches induced by a traumatic event activate intense and overwhelming emotions; these mismatches must be processed by way of assimilation and accommodation. Resick and Schnicke (1993) suggest that maladaptive assimilation and overaccommodation can occur, whereby the individual suffers from distorted thinking patterns and exaggerated changes to pre-existing schemata.

Also in a largely cognitive mould Horowitz (1973, 1974, 1979) has described an information processing model, one which underpins the structure of the Impact of Event Scale used in a number of studies of PTSD after illness. Emphasis is placed on processing of incoming information, and on cognitive theories of emotion; traumatic events involve massive amounts of internal and external information, most of which cannot be matched with current schemata since by their nature they are outside the realms of normal experience. Major elements of the model include information overload, incomplete information processing, and a 'completion tendency' where information must be processed repeatedly until reality and cognitive models match. This requires repeated attempts to process the raw data, thus traumatic information breaks through repeatedly, as evidenced by reports of intrusive, uncontrollable thoughts and vivid flashbacks or nightmares. This notion of a shattering of constructs as proposed by researchers like Janoff-Bulman and Horowitz may be helpful in understanding post-traumatic stress in ICU survivors. Except for the few cases where patients are undergoing readmission to the ICU, for very many patients admission and treatment may be cognitively disruptive in the extreme and have the potential to be very stressful. The information processing model may throw light on the experiences of these surviving patients.

Freud (1919) viewed military trauma from his own psychodynamic perspective, proposing that trauma to the psyche was a result of over-excitation of the individual's drives. Taking a very specific yet still essentially psychoanalytic view, Grubrich-Simitis (1987) considered the weight of stressors alongside the constitution of sufferers. These stressors included, among others, such things as disruption from family and usual environment, separation anxiety, helplessness and anticipation of death, annihilation of individuality and elimination of privacy. This may be somewhat esoteric, but it does not take a huge mental leap to translate some of these stressors to situations endured by some patients in the ICU, though of course there is no malevolent intent, and staff are striving to optimise wellbeing and reduce stress for patients. Separation anxiety occurs in those close to the critically ill patient, as a manifestation of loss and anticipatory grief – the natural and overwhelming fear in this situation is that the much loved individual may die. Yet separation anxiety may also occur in the sick patient who either recovers, or never loses, consciousness. Attachment figures may well appear to be lost to the patient, particularly when visiting is intermittent, analgesic drugs are causing confusion, and constant treatments or procedures are disrupting the patient's and relative's time together.

Sources of PTSD

Traumatic incidents like traffic accidents, violent attacks, and of course military or terrorist incidents, may be at the root of PTSD. But PTSD-related symptoms have also been demonstrated in other groups, for example in women following traumatic childbirth (Olde et al. 2006), and in patients following a range of experiences related to acute or critical illness; indeed being diagnosed with life-threatening disease has been recognised by the DSM-IV as a source of trauma. Cancer, as a life-threatening disease, is a source of interest for PTSD research (Jacobsen et al. 1998; Smith et al. 1999; Kwekkeboom and Seng 2002). Experiences related include reliving the time and hearing of diagnosis, painful procedures, bleeding, severe infections, side effects of treatment such as nausea and vomiting, and emotionally distressing associated events such as the response of family.

PTSD following discharge from ICU

Traumatic and violent incidents themselves may of course lead to intensive care admission. Yet as we have seen, the ICU experience *per se* has the potential to be quite stressful, and it has been suggested that some patients may fulfil criteria for PTSD after discharge from intensive care (Hall-Smith et al. 1997; Koshy et al. 1997; Schelling et al. 1998; Nickel et al. 2004). Schelling's study examined outcomes of adult acute respiratory distress syndrome (ARDS) including responses of patients nursed on high frequency 'jet' ventilators. Schelling suggested links between trauma endured in the ICU – acute anxiety, awareness of severe respiratory insufficiency, intrusive and repetitive ventilation noise, hallucinations and nightmares during treatment – and long-lasting effects on emotional wellbeing. The majority of survivors examined in this study reported only a moderate degree of physical impairment, yet a high frequency of significant psychosocial impairment. The reported incidence of PTSD in the ARDS survivors – 27.5% – was significantly higher than that in a control group. However we must remember that a feature of ARDS is profound hypoxaemia, raising susceptibility to cerebral hypoxic damage, which may sit alongside the ICU experience as a factor in psychological sequelae; cognitive impairment in ARDS survivors has been demonstrated in other groups (Hopkins et al. 1999, 2006).

It is clear that acute and critical illness can impact upon the psychological wellbeing of individuals. Across the UK a number of hospitals have established intensive care follow-up clinics where surviving patients can be assessed on a multidisciplinary basis, with attention paid to all aspects of physical recovery. At the same time psychological recovery can be explored, including the presence of any anxiety or depression, of PTSD-related symptoms, cognitive and psychosocial function. The approach is not fully consistent yet but this kind of support is a positive move in the overall care of the critically ill.

Conclusion

- Acute or critical illness can impact upon the psychological wellbeing of individuals, and the effects may last for some time.
- Information about the patient's psychological state is an important adjunct to information about clinical state.
- This chapter has examined aspects of acute and critical illness, along with certain psychological concepts which may help to explain

particular responses or outcomes. It is hoped this may help the practitioner to gain a fuller picture of the experience of the acutely ill patient, whether treated in a dedicated unit or not.

References

Abram H.S. (1965) Adaptation to open heart surgery: a psychiatric study of response to threat of death. *American Journal of Psychiatry* 122(9): 659–68.

American Psychiatric Association (APA) (1994) *Diagnostic and Statistical Manual of Mental Disorders*, 4th Edition. Washington DC: American Psychiatric Association.

Ashworth P. (1980) *Care to Communicate: an investigation into the problems of communication between patients and nurses in intensive therapy units.* RCN Research Series. London: Scutari Press.

Ashworth P. (1984) Communication in an intensive care unit. In A. Faulkner (ed.) *Communication.* Edinburgh: Churchill Livingstone.

Ashworth P. (1990) High technology and humanity for intensive care. *Intensive Care Nursing* 6(3): 150–60.

Bently S., Murphy F. and Dudley H. (1977) Perceived noise in surgical wards and in ICU. *British Medical Journal* 2(6101): 1503–6.

Brady J.V., Porter R., Conrad D. and Mason J. (1958) Avoidance behaviour and the development of gastroduodenal ulcers. *Journal of the Experimental Analysis of Behaviour* 1: 69–72.

Brewin C., Dalgleish T. and Joseph S. (1996) A dual representation theory of post traumatic stress disorder. *Psychological Review* 103: 670–86.

Cantor N., Norem J., Langston C. et al. (1991) Life tasks and daily life experiences. *Journal of Personality* 59(3): 425–51.

Cheng E. (1996) Recall in the sedated ICU patient. *Journal of Clinical Anaesthesia* 8: 675–78.

Coulter M.A. (1989) Needs of family members of patients in ICUs. *Intensive Care Nursing* 5(1): 4–10.

Devlin J., Fong J., Fraser G. and Riker R. (2007) Delirium assessment in the critically ill. *Intensive Care Medicine* 33(6): 929–40.

Dracup K. (1988) Are critical care units hazardous to health? *Applied Nursing Research* 1(1): 14–21.

Dyer I. (1995) Preventing the ITU syndrome or how not to torture an ITU patient! *Intensive and Critical Care Nursing* 11: 130–39.

Dyson M. (1999) Intensive care unit psychosis, the therapeutic nurse–patient relationship and the influence of the intensive care setting: analyses of interrelating factors. *Journal of Clinical Nursing* 8(3): 284–90.

Engel G.L. (1971) Sudden and rapid death during psychological stress. *Annals of Internal Medicine* 74: 771–82.

Engstrom A., Soderberg S. (2004) Experiences of partners of critically ill persons in an ICU. *Intensive and Critical Care Nursing* 20(5): 299–308.

Epstein S. (1990) Beliefs and symptoms in maladaptive resolution of the traumatic neurosis. In D. Ozer (ed.) *Perspectives on Personality* Vol. 3. London: Jessica Kingsley.

Fisher S. (1984) *Stress and the Perception of Control*. New Jersey, Lawrence Erlbaum Associates.

Freud S. (1919) *Introduction to the Psychology of the War Neuroses*. In Standard Edition 18, translated by J. Strachey. London: Hogarth Press.

Goldberger L. (1986) Sensory deprivation and overload. In Goldberger, Breznitz (eds.) *Handbook of Stress*. New York: Macmillan Press.

Grubrich-Simitis I. (1987) (ed.) Freud 1856–1939. A Phylogenetic Fantasy: Overview of the Transference Neuroses. Cambridge, MA: Bellknap Press of Harvard University Press.

Hagh-Shenas H., Goldstein L. and Yule W. (1999) Psychobiology of post traumatic stress disorder. In: W. Yule (ed.) *Post Traumatic Stress Disorders: Concepts and Therapy*. Chichester: Wiley.

Hall-Smith J., Ball C. and Coakley J. (1997) Follow up services and the development of a clinical nurse specialist in intensive care. *Intensive and Critical Care Nursing* 13: 243–8.

Hewitt P.B. (1970) Subjective follow-up of patients from a surgical intensive therapy ward. *British Medical Journal* 4(5736): 669–73.

Holland C., Cason C. and Prater L. (1997) Patients' recollections of intensive care. *Dimensions of Critical Care Nursing* 16: 132–41.

Holmes T.H. and Rahe R.H. (1967) The social readjustment rating scale. *Journal of Psychosomatic Research* 11: 213–8.

Hopkins R., Weaver L., Pope D., Orme J. and Bigler E. (1999) Neuropsychological sequelae and impaired health status in survivors of severe acute respiratory distress syndrome. *American Journal of Respiratory and Critical Care Medicine* 160(1): 50–6.

Hopkins R., Gale S. and Weaver L. (2006) Brain atrophy and cognitive impairment in survivors of acute respiratory distress syndrome. *Brain Injury* 20(3): 263–71.

Hopkinson R. and Freeman J. (1988) Therapeutic progress in intensive care, sedation and analgesia. *Journal of Clinical Pharmacy and Therapeutics* 13(1): 33–40.

Horne J. (1988) *Why we Sleep*. Oxford: Oxford University Press.

Horowitz M. (1973) Phase-oriented treatment of stress response syndromes. *American Journal of Psychotherapy* 27: 506–15.

Horowitz M. (1974) Stress response syndromes: character style and dynamic psychotherapy. *Archives of General Psychiatry* 31: 768–81.

Horowitz M. (1979) Psychological responses to serious life events. In V. Hamilton and D. Warburton (eds) *Human Stress and Cognition*. New York: Wiley.

Jacobsen P., Widows M. and Hann D. Posttraumatic stress disorder symptoms after bone marrow transplantation for breast cancer. *Psychosomatic Medicine* 60(3): 366–71.

Janoff-Bulman R. (1985) The aftermath of victimisation: rebuilding shattered assumptions. In C. Figley (ed.) Trauma and its wake – the study and treatment of PTSD. New York: Brunner Mazel.

Janoff-Bulman R. (1989) Assumptive worlds and the stress of traumatic events: applications the schema construct. *Social Cognition* 7(2): 113–36.

Jones C. and O'Donnell C. (1994) After intensive care – what then? *Intensive and Critical Care Nursing* 10: 89–92.

Jones C., Humphris G., Griffiths R. (1998) Psychological morbidity following critical care – the rationale for care after intensive care. *Clinical Intensive Care* 9: 199–205.

Jones C., Griffiths R., Humphris G. and Skirrow P. (2001) Memory, delusions and development of PTSD related symptoms after intensive care. *Critical Care Medicine* 29(35): 73–80.

Keane T., Fairbank J. and Caddell R. (1985) A behavioural approach to assessing and treating PTSD in Vietnam veterans. In C. Figley (ed.) *Trauma and its Wake*. New York: Brunner Mazel.

Kornfeld D. (1969) Psychiatric view of the intensive care unit. *British Medical Journal* 1(636): 108–10.

Koshy G., Wilkinson A., Harmsworth A. and Waldmann C. (1997) Intensive Care Unit follow up programme at a district general hospital. *Intensive Care Medicine* 23: 160.

Kwekkeboom K. and Seng J. (2002) Recognising and responding to PTSD in people with cancer. *Oncology nursing forum online* 29(4): 643–50.

Lovallo W.R. (1997) *Stress and Health: Biological and Psychological Interactions*. London: Sage Publications.

Lazarus R. (1966) *Psychological Stress and the Coping Process*. New York: McGraw-Hill.

Lazarus R. (1981) The stress and coping paradigm. In C. Eisdorfer, D. Cohen, A. Kleinman, and P. Maxim (eds) *Models for Clinical Psychopathology*. New York: Spectrum.

Lazarus R. (1999) *Stress and Emotion*. London: Springer.

Lazarus R.S. and Folkman S. (1984) *Stress, Appraisal and Coping*. New York: Springer.

Marks D., Murray M., Evans B. and Willig C. (2000) *Health Psychology: Theory, Research and Practice*. London: Sage.

McKegney F. (1966) The intensive care syndrome. *Connecticut Medicine* 30: 633–6.

Mills S. and Prough D. (1991) Neuropsychiatric complications following cardiac surgery. *Seminar Thoracic Cardiovascular Surgery* 3(1): 39–46.

Mittelman M.A., Maclure M. and Sherwood J. (1995) Triggering of acute myocardial infarction by episodes of anger. *Circulation* 92: 1720–5.

Molter N. (1979) Needs of relatives of critically ill patients. *Heart Lung* 8: 332–9.

Pervin L. (1989) Goal concepts in personality and social psychology: a historical perspective. In L. Pervin (ed.) *Goal Concepts in Personality and Social Psychology*. New Jersey, Laurence Erlbaum Associates.

National Institute for Health and Clinical Excellence (NICE) (2007) Acutely ill patients in hospital: recognition of and response to acute illness in adults in hospital. *NICE Clinical Guidelines* 50. www.nice.org.uk/CG050.

Nickel M., Leiberich P., Nickel C., Tritt K., Mitterlehner F., Rother W. and Loew T. (2004) The occurrence of posttraumatic stress disorder in patients following intensive care treatment: a cross-sectional study in a random sample. *Journal of Intensive Care Medicine* 19(5): 285–90.

Olde E., van der Hart O., Kleber R. and van Son M. (2006) Posttraumatic stress following childbirth. *Clinical Psychology Review* 26: 1–16.

Peterson C. and Seligman M.E.P. (1984) Causal explanations as a risk factor for depression: theory and evidence. *Psychological Review* 91: 347–74.

Pitman R. (1997) Overview of biological theories in PTSD. *Annals of New York Academy of Science* 821: 1–9.

Pun B. and Ely E. (2007) The importance of diagnosing and managing ICU delirium. *Chest* 132(2): 624–36.

Raps C., Peterson C., Jonas M. and Seligman M. (1982) Patient behaviour in hospitals: helplessness, reactance, or both? *Journal of Personality and Social Psychology* 42(6): 1036–41.

Resick P. and Schnicke M. (1993) Cognitive processing therapy for rape victims: a treatment manual. London: Sage Publications.

Rotter J. (1966) Generalised expectancies for internal versus external control of reinforcement. *Psychological Monographs* 80: 1–28.

Scheier M. and Carver C. (1987) Dispositional optimism and physical wellbeing: the influence of generalised outcome expectancies on health. *Journal of Personality* 55(2): 169–210.

Schelling G., Stoll C., Haller M., Briegel J., Manert W., Hummel T., Lenhart A., Heyduck M., Polasek J., Meier M., Preuss V., Bullinger M., Schuffel W. and Peter K. (1998) Health related quality of life and PTSD in survivors of acute respiratory distress syndrome. *Critical Care Medicine* 26(4): 651–9.

Seligman M.E., Maier S. and Solomon R.L. (1971) Unpredictable and uncontrollable aversive events. In F.R. Brush (ed.) *Aversive Conditioning and Learning*. New York: Academic Press.

Selye H. (1956) *The Stress of Life*. New York: McGraw-Hill.

Siegel L. and Peterson L. (1980) Stress reduction in young dental patients through coping skills and sensory information. *Journal of Consulting and Clinical Psychology* 48: 785–7.

Simpson-Wilson V. (1987) Identification of stressors related to patients' psychologic responses to the surgical ICU. *Heart Lung* 16(3): 267–73.

Smith M., Redd W., Peyser C. and Vogl D. (1999) Post-traumatic stress disorder in cancer: a review. *Psycho-Oncology* 8(6): 21–37.

Solomon P., Leiderman P. and Mendelson J. (1957) Sensory deprivation: a review. *American Journal of Psychology* 114: 357–63.

Stewart A. and Salt P. (1981) Life stress, lifestyles, depression and illness in adult women. *Journal of Personality and Social Psychology* 40(6): 1063–9.

Strahan E. and Brown R. (2005) A qualitative study of the experiences of patients following transfer from intensive care. *Intensive and Critical Care Nursing* 21(3): 160–71.

Taylor K. (1982) Brain damage during open heart surgery. *Thorax* 37: 873–6.

Thiagajaran J., Taylor P., Hogbin E. and Ridley S. (1994) Quality of life after multiple trauma requiring intensive care. *Anaesthesia* 49(3): 211–8.

Topf M., Bookman M. and Arand D. (1996) Effects of critical care unit noise on the subjective quality of sleep. *Journal of Advanced Nursing* 24: 545–51.

Weinman J., Johnston M. and Molloy G. (2006) *Health Psychology*. London: Sage.

Weiss J.M. (1970) Somatic effects of predictable and unpredictable shock. *Psychosomatic Medicine* 32: 397–408.

Weiss J.M. (1971) Effects of coping behaviour in different warning-signal conditions on stress pathology in rats. *Journal of Comparative and Physiological Psychology* 77: 1–13.

Wilkinson P. (1995)A qualitative study to establish the self-perceived needs of family members of patients in a general intensive care unit. *Intensive and Critical Care Nursing* 1995 11(2): 77–86.

Wortman C., Sheedy C., Gluhoski V. and Kessler R. (1992) Stress, coping and health: conceptual issues and directions for future research. In H. Friedman (ed.) *Hostility, Coping and Health*. Washington DC: American Psychological Association.

Chapter 3
Chronic illness

Jenny Waite-Jones

This chapter considers long-term illness, with particular emphasis on the bio-psycho-social nature of health and illness, as social status and related psychological processes have a profound impact on health. The social context of chronic illness is explored in terms of health inequalities, and links are demonstrated between stress and chronic illness through reference to psychoneuroimmunology and loss and adjustment, including lifestyle changes. Management strategies are considered with particular attention given to current initiatives within the National Health Service, including self help strategies such as patient led self-management programmes, and the extent to which 'patients' voices' are evident within current healthcare provision.

Adopting a bio-psycho-social approach to chronic illness helps avoid the fragmented, mechanistic approach of past medical services, and appreciates the 'person in context' (Trilling 2000). For example, heart disease may be biologically based, due to a genetic heart defect, but low economic status and related lack of education may lead to an unhealthy diet, obesity and strain on an already impaired heart. Halligan (2007) believes that social and cultural issues explain the gulf between illness presentation and disability better than traditional medical interpretations. Adopting a bio-psycho-social approach to chronic illness involves awareness of how the way society is structured influences individual behaviour. This can be conceptualised in terms suggested by Bronfenbrenner (1979). See Figure 3.1.

Bronfenbrenner's (1979; 2005) bio-ecological, systems-based approach helps to understand an individual's health experiences in terms of the systems within their family and wider society. This model

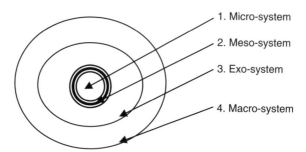

1. Micro-system
2. Meso-system
3. Exo-system
4. Macro-system

Micro-system: Interactions with those who directly influence the individual, including family members, extended family, peers, education, workplace and healthcare workers.
Meso-system: Interactions between the different elements of the microsystem, and the extent to which these can be seen to be 'joined up'.
Exo-system: Indirect influences including the media, employment opportunities, political, legal, health, and welfare policies.
Macro-system: Attitudes, values and beliefs identifiable within a specific culture which underpin the policies made within the exo-system.

Bronfenbrenner also noted that the impact of these systems vary over time as the person develops, and cultural and historical changes occur, and referred to this process as a **chrono-system**

Figure 3.1 Model based on Bronfenbrenner's (1979) theory, illustrating different interacting social systems influencing an individual's experience of chronic illness.

resembles a Russian doll-like structure with individual relationships embedded in, and influenced by, wider social structures. An individual's biologically inherited system is influenced by experiences within a micro-system, created through relationships with immediate and extended family members, as well as peers and others with whom the person interacts directly.

The way the various components of the micro-system, in turn, interact creates a meso-system, which can also impact on an individual's experience of chronic illness. For example, demands of work and/or education may conflict with family commitments and healthcare appointments. Trying to meet these demands may mean less time to interact with peers and maintain a social support network. Such experiences are influenced by a further, exo-system, which includes health and welfare policies and media representation, which are dictated by societal beliefs about health and disability held within a broader macro-system.

This bio-ecological approach helps to explain how social circumstances influence biologically based inherited characteristics, as one layer of the model impacts upon the others. A further dynamic within this process can be seen, through a chrono-system, as biologically based vulnerability towards ill health faced by individuals as they develop through their life-span is also influenced by cultural and historical changes at a macro level. For example, older age brings greater risks of heart disease and cancer, but the extent to which an individual may develop such conditions will be determined by the attitudes and lifestyle available to them through the cultural beliefs of the particular time in which they live.

British cultural norms and values allow inequalities in health experiences such that those from socially deprived areas, or marginalised groups, are more prone to, and adversely affected by, chronic ill health (Thomas and Dorling 2007). That an individual's experience of illness may be influenced by their socio-economic position, ethnicity, gender and related social structures (Peckham and Meerabeau 2007) needs to be considered when helping patients and clients adapt to the effects of chronic illness and disability.

Social context of chronic illness

When considering chronic illness it is important to appreciate that an individual's health beliefs are influenced by relationships within their family and peer group as well as the values of their community and wider society (Halligan 2007). Current improved life expectancy, due to improved disease control, means that such attitudes will impact on a greater number of people, as more are now likely to be living with chronic illness and disability than previously (Thomas and Dorling 2007). Moreover, those with a chronic illness are likely to develop new disabilities as they approach older age.

There is, thus, a need for many more individuals to manage their conditions and reduce disability, but the extent to which a person can do this may be determined by their social position including class, gender and ethnicity (Peckham and Meerabeau 2007). The gap between socio-economic groups and ill health continues to increase within Britain, and major 'cultural' changes in thinking and behaviour are required to reduce this discrepancy (Marmot and Wilkinson 2001).

Class, gender and ethnicity and chronic illness

Links between chronic illness and class were apparent in the 1980s when the Black Report (see Townend et al. 1992) suggested that, at all stages of life, those belonging to lower social classes had worse health. For example, twice as many men, and two and half times more women in class 5 (unskilled manual) reported having a chronic illness than class 1 (professional). The Acheson Report (1998) also found longstanding illness to be influenced by inequalities in terms of socio-economic status, ethnicity and gender. Sadly, such inequalities still exist in the 21st century. Thomas and Dorling (2007) link chronic illness to low socio-economic status, and Marmot and Wilkinson (2001) relate low socio-economic position, racism and discrimination against women to current health inequalities.

Bosna et al. (1999) found that, even, adverse socio-economic conditions early in childhood can affect later adult ill health, including cardiovascular conditions, severe heart conditions and strokes. Socio-economic disadvantage has been linked to onset and progression of disability of patients diagnosed with rheumatoid arthritis (Grundy and Glaser 2000), and higher mortality rates for those with this condition (Maiden, et al. 1999). Moreover, having rheumatoid arthritis increases relative poverty and lack of access to services.

Poor health within some ethnic groups has also been related to poverty, racism, and lack of education (Marmot and Wilkinson 2001). Individuals whose family are of Pakistani and Bangladeshi origin are more likely to suffer unemployment, poverty and ill health (Peckham and Meerabeau 2007) and feel socially disadvantaged through lack of understanding of how their religious beliefs impact upon their condition (Rhodes et al. 2008). Also, Feder et al. (2002) found that, whilst prone to coronary disease, Asian patients were less likely to undergo coronary bypass operations, possibly due to socio-economic, cultural and language difficulties. In addition, Peckham and Meerabeau (2007) report high levels of poverty and ill health amongst other ethnic groups, such as migrant workers and asylum seekers, but explain difficulties in assessing the true extent of this relationship due to their non-resident status.

Women report more illness and are more likely to have a chronic condition yet live longer than men. Such differences in chronic illness may be due to female socialisation, as gender role expectations are embedded within social structures and can create different lifestyles and behaviour (Nettleton 2000). Women may be more vulnerable to chronic conditions because of having to take on multiple roles and experience economic disadvantage, low status at work, being responsible for the care of others and budgeting on low income (Peckham and Meerabeau 2007). For example, Treharne et al. (2007) report women are more likely than men to suffer depression and arthritis, and have less perceived control.

Moreover, whilst many more men than women have heart related conditions, Plach (2008) found that women are more likely to be hospitalised later due to complications, report a lower quality of life, be more prone to diabetes and hypertension, and twice as likely to be disabled than men.

Explanations for links between class, ethnicity and gender and chronic illness

When considering links between ill health and socio-economic position, ethnicity and gender it is always possible that data collection and classification techniques may be open to different interpretations. For example, different systems may be used to measure socio-economic status, and ethnic group may be defined through self-classification or ascribed by an interviewer. Also, gender differences in terms of higher female morbidity may be based on self-report studies and males may be less likely to report ill health. Findings may, also, be specific to particular geographical areas rather than the population as a whole.

Furthermore, 'social selection' could be used to explain how ill health may actually determine socio-economic status, and biologically inherited conditions common to some ethnic groups may create social disadvantage. For example, anaemia, diabetes and schizophrenia are more common amongst Afro-Caribbean descendents and cerebrovascular disease and diabetes are some of the conditions most prevalent in those of Asian descent (Porter et al. 1999). Also, biological difference between the sexes may explain some gender differences and ill health as, for example, hormonal links could explain, at least to some extent, the high number of women with rheumatoid arthritis.

Nevertheless, Davey Smith et al. (2001) state that 'social selection' can only contribute in a minor way to explaining current health inequalities. Also, Marmot and Wilkinson (2001) suggest that, despite some potential difficulties regarding data classification, enough evidence exists to suggest that health inequalities are due to material factors and related lifestyle behaviours, which need to be tackled at a social/structural level. They cite, poor living conditions, lack of achievement in the education system, poor employment opportunities and negative attitudes and treatment as stressful, and impacting on health.

Lynch et al. (2000) see poverty as the cause of health inequalities, and suggest that offering psychosocial explanations may imply that an individual's lifestyle is more to blame. They feel that this latter explanation allows governments to avoid their responsibility for making changes at a structural level, and leads to scapegoating individuals, who are powerless to do otherwise within the existing social structures. However, Marmot and Wilkinson (2001) disagree, arguing that the interrelatedness of psychosocial and structural/ material factors needs to be considered to fully understand continuing inequalities in health.

Having a low income may increase difficulties in coping with the loss of previous good health and this also may be reacted to differently in terms of age, gender and ethnicity. For example, Kiviruusu et al. (2007) found more young males than females with diabetes, asthma and migraine to suffer depression. The extent to which autonomy and independence are valued at a macro-level within British society makes it difficult for individuals to express grief for such loss (Field and Payne 2003) and adjust to the level of dependence required by particular chronic illnesses.

Social attitudes, self-esteem and chronic illness

Values and beliefs regarding illness and disability within the macro-system can influence how chronic illness is experienced at an individual level. For example, Smith and Osborn (2007) found that patients with chronic low back pain felt constantly judged by others, and that struggling to fulfil their social roles was more stressful than the pain created by their condition. Bury (2001: 227) suggests that even healthcare professionals 'marginalize the existential dimension' of patients' experiences. He says that a truly holistic approach in healthcare requires acknowledging patients' beliefs, lifestyle and circumstances as well as recognising the 'ecology of relationships in which they are embedded' within a particular cultural setting.

Marmot and Wilkinson (2001: 234) state that in Britain 'wealth makes for social status, success, and respectability – just as poverty is stigmatising' and, as chronic illness and disability compounds a person's low income this may lead to labelling and social exclusion. Labelling, based on judgements of what is seen as 'normal' or 'deviant' within society, includes primary deviance, the actual illness or disability defined as 'deviant', and secondary deviance, the way people react to the label (Lemert 1972). However, secondary deviance may result in stereotyping and self-fulfilling prophecies of those ascribed labels. For example, as a person with a chronic illness and disability is expected to be passive and accept offers of help with gratitude, those with heart related conditions may begin to see themselves as less than normal or inferior and fear taking exercise or going back to work, particularly if they had a manual job.

Moreover, labels based on particular conditions can be embarrassing and, although ascribed by others, become part of the patient's identity. Bury (2001) offers an example of a patient who struggled to maintain a sense of self-worth after embarrassing bowel surgery and refused to be labelled an 'ileostomist'. Sapey (2001) describes how medical professionals, overly concerned with bodily dysfunctions, are ever ready to medicalise behaviour and ascribe appropriate labels. This brings to mind a personal experience of feeling compelled to reply to a colleague, when he disclosed that he was a 'bruxer', 'You are just a person who grinds your teeth!'

However, as Sapey (2001) points out, medical labels can also bring benefits. Having a label ascribed to a set of behaviours can be a relief and absolve the patient, their family, and others from a sense of responsibility. For example, once a child is given the label attention deficit hyperactivity disorder (ADHD) parents and teachers can feel their skills are no longer questioned, have the child statemented and receive financial help. Nevertheless, the emotional and financial befts of disease diagnosis may be outweighed if disabled people are unable to apply for a mortgage or receive insurance coverage (Smith 2002). Also, ambiguous attitudes at governmental level have meant improved public disability awareness whilst claiming benefits has become increasingly more difficult (Sapey 2001).

Thus, explanations of health inequalities also have to consider individuals' perception of their experiences, which in turn are influenced by their social context. That stress is related to lifestyle, structural constraints and chronic illness is evident in the findings of Marmot et al.'s (1984, 1991) studies of civil servants. Heart disease was seen as linked to lack of autonomy, variety, direction or control, with job dissatisfaction influencing increased sickness absences. Marmot et al. suggest that health inequalities are created by stress due to environmental factors and individuals' perception of their relative position within an occupational and social hierarchy.

Marmot and Wilkinson (2001: 234) demonstrate how, at a broader societal level, the lower the class gradient a worker is in, the less control and variety they experience at work. They also show how women are much more likely to experience such restrictions and monotony than men. However, although severe lack of social support was also more prevalent as the social class gradient decreased, women were less likely to experience this to the same extent as men in the same social class category. (The relationship between social support and ill health will be discussed later in this chapter). Marmot and Wilkinson (2001: 234) conclude that 'relative deprivation involving control over life, insecurity, anxiety, social isolation, socially hazards environments, bullying and depression' are linked to people's position within socio-economic structures, and demonstrate how psychosocial factors are related to ill health such as heart disease.

Bury (2001) found that people with heart conditions clearly understood that, although their illness may be due to an inherited predisposition, social conditions and environment were also influential. Structural inequalities may undermine a person's 'just beliefs', which are based on a sense of social equality. Experiencing social inequalities when equality is expected can undermine their sense of self-worth and identity (Lucas et al. in press). Feeling unfairly treated can lead to feeling stressed, and related health-risky coping behaviour, such as smoking, alcohol consumption, lack of exercise and comfort eating.

Stress may be seen as both precipitating, and compounded by, chronic illness. Providing effective healthcare for those with a chronic illness thus requires understanding not only the social context of patients but also their perceptions of their social and individual position, and the level of control they feel that they have over their lives.

Stress and chronic illness

Most doctors now acknowledge potential links between stress and any disease (Hippisley-Cox et al. 1998). However, identifying and defining stress is complex, as this transaction between the mind and body includes biologically based characteristics interacting with the way an individual perceives their situation, and may be modified by the particular coping strategies they adopt.

Stress has been linked to a number of chronic conditions, such as dermatological disorders and particularly psoriasis (Evers et al. 2005; Vargas et al. 2006). Hennessy et al. (2001) demonstrated a biological basis of stress in animals suffering maternal separation. They exhibited 'despair' and 'sickness behaviour' similar to human depression which was accompanied by impaired immune functioning. Depression, an increasingly common chronic condition in itself, is also linked to other disorders such as rheumatoid arthritis (Treharne et al. 2007). Hippisley-Cox et al. (1998) point out that depression may accompany symptoms of ischaemic heart disease, and Sheehy et al. (2006) suggest that new biological treatments for rheumatoid arthritis may prove useful in reducing depression as well as inflammation.

Anxiety, also associated with stress, can accompany depression (Campo et al. 2004). Vandyke et al. (2004) found anxiety and depression prevalent in patients with rheumatoid arthritis, and suggested measuring these separately as they can vary. Different forms of anxiety have been found linked to specific disorders: patients with neurological, vascular and respiratory conditions exhibited simple phobias; gastrointestinal, metabolic and autoimmune conditions were related to social phobias; and heart disease was linked to panic attacks and agoraphobia (Sareen et al. 2005). Treating the anxiety may help reduce illness symptoms.

The biological basis of stress

Anxiety and depression can be determined by the amount of stimulation a person experiences and, thus, demonstrates the extent to which the body is a complex, self-regulating system. Too much and too little stimulation can create a stress response (Frankenhaeuser 1980). Apter (1997) suggests that emotional states, and their role in achieving goals are complex; anxiety and depression may impede a person's ability to carry out general tasks as well as the constant negotiations created by chronic illness.

Selye (1956) extended work established by Cannon (1929) and developed the theory of a 'general adaptation syndrome' to explain biological reactions to stress. This suggests that the immediate response to the impact of a stressor is an increase in the release of adrenaline and endorphins, to facilitate 'fight or flight'. Whilst resistance is then maintained through the release of cortisol, over time the production of these, and other related chemical changes, compromise the immune system and may leave the stressed person susceptible to disease. Such a system may have evolved in response to life-threatening physical dangers, but in current, technologically based, Western society psychologically stressful experiences increasingly influence health, particularly in relation to chronic stress and the immune system.

Psychoneuroimmunology

'There is now absolutely no doubt in scientific circles that psychological experiences can influence the activity of our immune systems' (Evans et al. 1997: 303) and current work in psychoneuroimmunology offers exciting new ways of understanding the 'mind/body' relationship in terms of stress. Bi-directional pathways between the brain and immune system, and related immunological changes mediate psychological effects of some diseases. For example, chronic, unrelenting stress has been associated with down regulation of the immune system and reduced activity of natural killer cells which play an important role in fighting malignant disease (Kiecolt-Glaser 1999).

However, whilst a possible relationship exists between stress and chronic health conditions, such as cancer and rheumatoid arthritis, it is very difficult to quantify stress. Reactions to a particular event can vary between people, and even the same individual may react differently to the same event, at different times, according to a range of personal and situational factors. Nevertheless, studies have demonstrated how some common critical life-events, such as bereavement, impact upon the immune system as it strives to achieve a balance between up and down regulation (Evans et al. 1997).

Phillips and Burns (2008: 302) explain how cells within the immune system 'tag, destroy or neutralize, bacterial, viruses or other harmful or foreign material (antigens)' and that antibody levels are 'a result of a culmination of a series of immunological events, starting with "foreign body" antigen recognition, and resulting in the production of very specific antibodies by B cells'. They used vaccines to mimic illness processes in an attempt to determine which cells within the immune system may be susceptible and found those specifically related to T cells as influential within the stress process. Whilst results from short-term stress ('challenging' tasks given prior to immunisation) suggested an initial positive immune response to stress, participants who had suffered bereavement within the previous year produced less antibodies after vaccination. However, Phillips and Burns (2008) also found that the person's age and the severity of stress may be influential, particularly as the immune system is less effective in older age.

Links between stress and chronic illness are particularly complex as the chemical changes resulting from chronic, unrelenting stress including daily inconveniences, can create an impaired or overactive immune system, leaving the stressed individual prone to specific kinds of illness. Straub et al. (2005) explain that levels of perceived stress influence the levels of cortisol production, which in turn triggers a chain of complex chemical reactions. It would appear that the effects of some very specific levels of stress on cortisol production can prove immune suppressing, and create a susceptibility to cancer and infections, whilst cortisol production from other specific stress levels creates immunostimulation, which is linked to inflammatory conditions such as rheumatoid and juvenile arthritis.

The relationship between stress and cortisol production is particularly complicated as Straub et al. (2005: 21) suggest that chemical reactions within the inflammatory process create further changes within the immune system resulting in habituation to cortisol and a need for higher levels for this to be effective. Such an explanation helps in understanding the relationship between flare-ups and stressful events common in chronic, inflammatory conditions.

Personality and stress

Susceptibility to stress and related chronic illness has also been linked to personality traits, which may have a biological basis. A person's temperament, based on their inherited neurology, may determine the extent to which they respond to different levels of stimuli (Thomas and Chess 1977). For example, type A individuals, who are impatient and express feelings of anger and hostility, are thought to be at risk of coronary and arterial illness (Davidson et al. 2007). Neurotic, extrovert and pessimistic personalities have been associated with stress related illnesses (Ferguson et al. 1999; Phillips and Burns 2008), and Treharne et al. (2007) found personality styles to be linked to depression and inflammatory conditions.

However, whilst Ferguson et al. (1999) agree that personality traits such as neuroticism and extroversion are related to stress and illness, they point out that personality is an intimate relationship between cognition and emotion, which may have a biological basis, but also involves schemas constructed from past experiences which influence a person's appraisal and emotional response. For example, a pessimistic personality may result from repeated negative experiences, which, over time, create a tendency towards negative appraisal. This may become encoded in the person's self-schema and result in feelings of low self-esteem and self-worth and pessimism about new situations.

Cognitive explanations of stress

Current stress theories acknowledge cognitive explanations, such as those by Lazarus and Folkman (1984). This computational approach suggests that the judgements people make are based upon schemas they have developed from past experiences, which influence their perception of their present situation and how they should respond. Stress, thus, emerges from the gap between what people perceive is expected of them, and their ability to meet these demands. If the gap is small, the response required is perceived as a challenge, but if the gap is large it is felt to be stressful.

Ferguson et al. (1999) utilise Lazarus and Folkman's (1984) model in relation to chronic illness to explain how people initially judge situations as a threat (possibly physically harmful and anxiety provoking), a challenge (facilitating personal growth as informative and stimulating) or a loss (including suffering and potentially intolerable pain). Such judgements are seen as based, to some extent, on personality, and influencing health and coping behaviour.

Control, self-efficacy and learned helplessness

Stress, thus, appears to occur when individuals feel they are not in control of their situation, and may through related immunological changes precipitate chronic illness. Such illness also reduces the amount of control a person has over many aspects of their life. The level of control people feel they have has been found to impact upon their health related behaviour. Rotter (1966) differentiated between people who display an internal locus of control, through believing they were able to control events, and those exhibiting an external locus of control, through believing that events were either controlled by other people or forces within their environment. Abramson et al. (1978) later demonstrated the need to consider the extent to which individuals may assess events as under their control or outside their control at some times, but not others (stable versus unstable) and in all ways or only in certain situations (global versus specific).

The extent to which a person feels they are in control can influence their health beliefs and related behaviour, as those with an internal locus of control believe their actions can change situations and will seek information and actively take care of their health. However, those with an external locus of control see their health as beyond their control, that luck, fate or chance is responsible for their situation, and that others are unlikely to be able to help. Those with this type of external view are less likely to behave in ways to promote health, prevent ill health or foster rehabilitation. Younger et al. (2007) suggest that symptoms of rheumatoid arthritis are both a cause and result of stress, and found a sense of control rather than fatalism helpful in managing related pain and fatigue.

A sense of control is also related to levels of self-efficacy (Bandura 1977): if individuals perceive some positive outcome resulting from their efforts they will increase their efforts to manage their condition, respond more productively to feedback and develop higher self-esteem. Those with a low sense of self-efficacy are likely to give up more easily and fail to use feedback to improve their condition. Lowe et al. (2007) found increased self-efficacy, and a sense of mastery, in rheumatoid arthritis patients who received positive feedback in relation to their own actions, or witnessed successful actions of other, similar patients. Lau-Walker (2006) also found increasing self-efficacy and changing illness representations helped patients experiencing cardiac rehabilitation.

In contrast, feeling a lack of control and experiencing limited opportunities to develop self-efficacy can lead to learned helplessness. Seligman and Maier's (1975) work suggested that those who feel that they cannot change the outcome of their situation cease trying to do so. Learned helplessness may result from uncontrollable positive as well as negative events if individuals have no opportunity to put any effort into achieving outcomes. For example, Kiviruusu et al. (2007) found that if those with a chronic illness are not allowed to feel some sense of responsibility for their care, they may cease trying to help themselves and experience feelings of helplessness, hopelessness, low self-esteem and depression. Such feelings may exacerbate existing limitations on an individual's social and professional life created by chronic illness, and mean less opportunity to develop social skills, control events or receive positive feedback for actions taken, and, thus, may increase feelings of learned helplessness.

Loss, adjustment and coping with chronic illness

Those with long-term health conditions can experience chronic sorrow through having to face recurring losses in terms of health and lifestyle. Experiences of loss were perceived by participants with rheumatoid arthritis to be related to the onset and flare-ups of their illness (Waite-Jones 1998), and families with a child with juvenile idiopathic arthritis reported a loss of normal family life (Waite-Jones 2005). The response to having a chronic illness can be seen as a form of bereavement requiring support and coping strategies to promote adjustment.

Reactions to chronic illness may include use of defence mechanism based on Freudian theory as pointed out by Folkman et al. (1986). For example, patients may suspect their previous smoking of causing cancer and displace their guilty feelings on to healthcare staff, accusing them of neglecting their care. Alternatively, patients may project their own negative attitudes towards disability on to others, and feel belittled by them. Such strategies may in turn have a negative effect on a patient's self-esteem and reinforce unconscious negative beliefs towards their condition.

Coping can be seen as an attempt to make unfavourable circumstances more favourable (Kovacs 2007) and helps tolerate experiences created by chronic illness. Coping strategies can help normalise and limit the effects of the illness on the patient's sense of personal identity, or allow the illness to become the patient's identity in an attempt to control situations through enhancing predictability. Coping becomes a complex mix of personal values, perceptions and beliefs embedded in social circumstances which are, to some extent, dictated by wider social structures (Bury 2001).

Coping strategies can be problem focused (active) and involve attempts to change difficult situations, or emotion focused and attempt to change the feelings created by such situations. The positive or negative effects of both kinds of strategies are determined by individual circumstances. Rather than seeing avoidance as a form of emotional coping, Moos and Holahan (2003) see it as a separate style and point out how it may have short-term benefits, but generally proves harmful long term. Kovacs (2007) also suggests avoidance can be seen as problematic if it just means avoiding facing stressful situations, but can prove adaptive if it means recognising and acting in a way which avoids creating stressful situations.

However, studies in psychoneuroimmunology suggest that links between coping styles, stress and immune function are complex. Active coping styles have been linked to positive changes in the immune system but only in terms of high level stress, whilst avoidance has a positive effect in response to low, but not high level stress (Stowell et al. 2001). Sheehy, Murphy and Barry (2006) found active coping most useful when patients were first diagnosed with rheumatoid arthritis, but Thompson et al. (2002) found those with vitiligo (a skin complaint) had to use a number of different strategies as, whilst problem solving was less problematic than avoidance, it was more difficult to sustain.

Social support

Social support offers the opportunity to confide in others, which helps in coping with chronic illness. Such support is not dependent upon the size of a person's network, but rather on how supportive relatives and friends are perceived to be. Larger social networks can bring further stress in terms of keeping in contact with a greater number of people, and caring about more people brings the risk of more loss over time (O'Donovan and Hughes 2006). If perceived as inappropriate, such support can have a negative effect, and even be felt to be a form of social control (Ryan et al. 2003).

Moos and Holahan (2003) suggest that perceived social support, particularly from family members, facilitates self-esteem and confidence in the face of overwhelming situations. They point out how it provides the opportunity to consider situations from another's perspective and receive feedback, which helps in assessing, planning and adopting more adaptive coping methods, as well as reducing avoidance and emotional discharge. They offer examples of depressed, male patients who tend to rely on alcohol if they have no family support, and female patients with rheumatoid arthritis who will adopt more cognitive strategies, including information seeking, if they have such support.

Phillips and Burns (2008) also found social support to mediate against immunological vulnerability to stress, with happily married couples exhibiting greater immune response than those who were single or in poor relationships. However, whilst Sherman et al. (2006) report social support as helpful in reducing depression but not improving physical health, Dekkers et al. (2001) found that such support can moderate pain to some extent.

A complex picture thus emerges when considering the relationship between stress and chronic illness, including interrelated systems determining how individual and environmental demands impact on health, but are also mediated by aspects of personality, developed from past experiences and particular coping strategies adopted, as well as factors specific to the situation faced at any particular point of a person's life (Moos and Holahan 2003). Helping those with a chronic condition involves recognising the complexity of this process, and encouraging them to develop proactive coping which includes: recognising potential stressors, initially appraising these, attempting and monitoring specific coping strategies and constructively using feedback (Kovacs 2007).

Managing chronic illness

From evidence offered so far within this chapter it can be seen that the extent to which stress impacts upon chronic illness is due to an individual's perception of their situation as well as their particular social context. Whilst the need for change at a social structural level, demanded by Lynch et al. (2000), is acknowledged, it is not possible in one chapter to suggest how health inequalities may be tackled. However, it is possible to consider individual behaviour and lifestyle, which Marmot and Wilkinson (2001) see is also necessary, and explore helpful ways of coping with stress related to chronic illness.

Health promotional strategies influencing changes in lifestyle to help avoid chronic illness can be implemented on both societal and individual levels. However, Bennett and Murphy (2001) point out that, whilst interventions targeting specific groups as well as the whole population have proved of some use in changing individual behaviour, health inequalities may continue to increase as it is usually well-educated, white collar workers who engage in health promoting behaviour. Caution is needed as, at an individual level, Senior et al. (2002) found that patients who were informed that they could have controlled the onset of their condition by behaving otherwise were reluctant to disclose their diagnosis to others, and held more negative feelings about themselves.

Although it not possible to avoid many stressful life events, and some level of stress is necessary to maintain sufficient arousal to carry out tasks, it is possible to help those with chronic illness to adopt strategies to cope with stress. Increasing feelings of control, self-efficacy and perceived social support to reduce the risk of learned helplessness are core principles within stress management and under-pin current interventions, including counselling, cognitive behavioural therapy and self-help strategies.

Therapeutic interventions

Counselling offered, informally and formally, within healthcare and voluntary groups, can be used as a focused intervention or accompany other therapeutic approaches. Good interpersonal skills, including listening, attending to verbal as well as non-verbal cues and displaying empathy, genuineness and unconditional positive regard (as advocated within humanistic psychology) help to develop supportive relationships (Nelson-Jones 2001). Such a relationship helps those with a chronic condition to develop the confidence, skills and self-efficacy required to make necessary life changes, and is particularly useful for those who have little perceived social support.

Expressive writing can also be useful in allowing those with chronic conditions to articulate their concerns and reflect upon their experiences. Smyth et al. (1999) noted improvements in patients with asthma and rheumatoid arthritis, who expressed their feelings in writing; Danoff-Burg et al. (2006) found expressive writing helpful for patients diagnosed with lupus erythematosus and rheumatoid arthritis; and Hamilton-West and Quine (2007) report some success in the use of expressive writing with patients who have ankylosing spondylitis. It appears that such writing helps develop the ability to cognitively restructure attitudes and appraise experiences more positively.

Cognitive behavioural therapy (CBT), widely used within current healthcare, attempts to increase feelings of control and self-efficacy and reduce feelings of helplessness. CBT involves adopting a collaborative approach, encouraging identification of concerns, gathering evidence to substantiate or refute beliefs upon which such concerns are based, and acting upon conclusions drawn. CBT attempts to enhance self-esteem and recognises links between mood and behaviour (Hawton et al. 1989). The aim is to break the cycle of dysfunctional thinking and related emotions that may have developed through struggling to come to terms with a disabling condition, for example, encouraging those avoiding physical activity after receiving cardiac surgery to engage in graded exercise and report back on how this felt.

Rhee et al. (2000) found CBT enhanced self-efficacy and positive coping as well as indirectly reduced pain and depression in patients with rheumatoid arthritis. Whilst CBT avoids the potential reactions and addiction associated with pharmacological therapies it is time consuming and needs trained staff, which can be costly short-term. However, long term, offering CBT may prove cost effective in reducing the use of other medical services. For example, Davidson et al. (2007) successfully used CBT to reduce hostility in patients with type A personalities and heart disease, and found this linked to direct reductions in hospital costs due to shorter length of inpatient stay and less medication or outpatient visits. They concluded that further, hidden long-term costs made this treatment a true investment.

Some techniques within CBT are used within, and alongside, other approaches, including patient education, cardiac rehabilitation programmes, pain management, relaxation, hypnosis and visual imaging. For example, hypnosis and relaxation help, through professional suggestion, to alter aspects of illness such as pain perception (Dixon et al. 2007). Such techniques have been found to improve immune response. For example, increased natural killer cell activity and other cellular changes were noted after use of relaxation by Kiecolt-Glaser (1999), and Castes et al. (1999) reported similar immunological changes when using relaxation and guided imaging with asthmatic children and also found these children to use less medication and experience fewer episodes of attacks than controls. Dixon et al. (2007) found CBT, emotional disclosure and hypnosis all to be useful in helping patients cope with chronic conditions, but CBT proved the most successful in relation to managing pain and learning adaptive coping skills.

Self-care, self-help and self-management

Self-care, self-help and self-management have been used interchangeably within published literature, yet self-care refers to health promoting behaviour used by any individual, whilst self-help relates to supportive strategies which can improve experiences of those living with a chronic condition (Barlow et al. 2005). Support groups promote self-help through increasing social support, providing positive role models and helpful tips for day-to-day living with chronic illness, as well as campaigning to change public attitudes. However, not all those with a chronic condition wish to associate with similar others and, on a practical level, such groups may suffer funding difficulties and be seen as a 'cheap alternative' to professional led services. Nevertheless, Moos and Holahan (2003) suggest that support groups can help ameliorate social and coping deficits, and cite Alcoholics Anonymous as more successful than outpatient care in reducing alcohol addiction. Barlow et al. (2005) also note how support groups are also increasingly offering education and advice.

Self-management, according to Barlow et al. (2005), adopts a purposefully instructive approach in relation to symptom control, treatment and psychosocial consequences on lifestyle, which compliments patient education offered by healthcare professionals. Whilst self-management strategies include some of the principles underpinning CBT it is often lay-led which, as well as encouraging participants to identify their individual needs and skills and increase in confidence, offers the opportunity for the course leader to be perceived as a guide and model.

A self-management programme which has proved particularly successful for patients diagnosed with arthritis was developed by Kate Lorig (see Barlow et al. 2000). The Arthritis Self Management Programme (ASMP) is a highly structured programme delivered over six weeks, based on a common manual and delivered by two lay-leaders who have arthritis themselves. Whilst Lorig found that professionals could run such programmes equally successfully, lay-leaders were preferred so as to offer role models and make the programme accessible through the voluntary sector. The charity Arthritis Care has achieved considerable success in delivering this programme.

The principles within the ASMP were later developed to become, the more generic, Chronic Disorder Self Management Programme (CDSM), which includes developing problem solving techniques, exercise, managing fatigue, sleeplessness, cognitive appraisal and problem solving, and emotional responses as well as information on nutrition, medication, community resources and ways of improving communication with professionals (Holman and Lorig 1997).

Positive responses to the CDSM have meant that a modified version now forms the basis of the Expert Patient Programme (EPP) offered within the National Health Service. A government report (DH 2000) outlined a six-year plan to introduce user led self-management programmes in England, to be available from all Primary Care Trusts (PCTs) by 2004. The EPP employs similar techniques to the CDSM, by means of a six-week course which is meant to be lay-led and aims to enhance patients' sense of control and ability to manage their condition, and help them develop skills and confidence to partner professionals in their own care. New initiatives since 2004 include offering EPPs to parents of children with chronic conditions, and since 2005 lay-led self-management programmes have become a major component of health policies in Britain (Newbould et al. 2006).

Donaldson (2003: 326) claims that the EPP helps utilise patients' own experiences so that a 'true partnership between the public and health professionals can be forged', empowering patients to become experts in their own care. However, Donaldson also acknowledges that for the EPP to be successful there needs to be a change in the attitudes of patients and health professionals.

Some success has been reported with such self-management programmes. For example, Buszewickz et al. (2006) found improved self-efficacy relating to symptom management of patients with osteoarthritis but no significant improvement on pain, physical function and use of primary care services, whilst Kuijer et al. (2007) found no effects regarding self-efficacy, or proactive coping but some positive physical effects in patients with asthma. Ockleford et al. (2008) report that people with type 2 diabetes preferred education and self-management programmes. Brooker et al. (2008) found people with type 1 diabetes felt more in control of their lives, valued the trustworthiness of information and regular contact with similar others possible through such programmes.

Nevertheless, Newbould et al. (2006) carried out a systematic review of lay-led self-management courses such as the EPP and found some short-term benefits, but felt that these had possibly been overstated as the varied experiences of those with different chronic conditions, including severe mental illness, made assessment difficult. Taylor and Bury (2007) found that recruitment to the EPP has been disappointing and Newbould et al. (2006) point out that reported success may due to participant bias, given the dominance of self-selected, well-educated females whose comments may reflect the positive response inherent within the 'coaching' of such courses. Rogers (2006) suggests this overstating may be due to the relative newness to the NHS of thinking underlying the EPP which includes the 'can do' attitude of the USA, and also that the NHS may feel compelled to justify the expense of having invested so heavily in this initiative.

In addition to information located from published literature, personal experiences of involvement with the early introduction and progress of ASMP, including attending a workshop run by Kate Lorig, have offered the opportunity to observe first hand some very positive effects of this programme on people with arthritis. Working with EPP lay-leaders has enabled an appreciation of some concerns with regard to the way this approach has been adopted within the NHS. Whilst successful when offered to condition-specific groups by Arthritis Care, the mix of conditions within the EPP appears to inhibit learning about specific conditions and related treatment as well as reduce the impact of social support from those with similar illness experiences.

Newbould et al. (2006) also point out that condition-specific self-management strategies already exist within communities, albeit in a piecemeal fashion. They warn against the EPP being seen as a 'pill for all ill', as not all patients wish to disclose their condition or even consider it to be chronically disabling. For example, patients with mild to moderate asthma may not be enthusiastic about EPP as they often find themselves having to deal with spasmodic episodes rather than having a chronic illness.

Whilst Battersby (2006) suggests that Newbould et al. (2006) are rather overcritical of such a new initiative as the EPP, Griffiths et al. (2007) see it as somewhat costly and feel that more evaluation is required to assess the extent to which it is offering value for money. Taylor and Bury (2007) are also cautious about the EPP in case it may be seen as a 'magic bullet' in comparison to the other, more costly and radical societal changes necessary. They fear that it may mask the need for social change, be offered at the expense of other services, and that concentrating on changing lifestyle could lead to blaming individuals living with a chronic illness is as much socially as medically defined.

Bury (2004) is concerned that the EPP should be seen as a single step in the larger process of patient care and not detract from voluntary initiatives or people's other preferred ways of managing their illness. Bury, like Finn (2006), sees such programmes as part of a pluralist response to helping manage chronic illness, including more egalitarian relationships between patients and professionals involved in their care.

Patient/professional partnerships

The EPP can be seen as part of a broader attempt to offer more appropriate healthcare provision for those with chronic conditions. Holman (2005, 2007) points out that current health services are based around acute rather than chronic provision. Caring for those with chronic conditions requires maximising comfort and function. Medicine and surgery may be required, but necessary skills also include the ability to initiate behaviour change and emotional adjustment in order to guide patients who are the principal care-givers. Holman (2005) suggests that a model of care based on chronic illness should include: educating and training patients and their family in self-management skills; team care including the patient as a member; creating and implementing a team management plan with defined roles and responsibilities; and evaluation of individual and group outcomes.

The need for such a shift in thinking within healthcare is identified in the NHS Executive document (DH 1997) concerning patient and professional partnerships. This document reports a need for improved communication from professionals and the development of a collaborative strategy between patients and healthcare professionals. Current organisational cultures within healthcare, and professionals' lack of appreciation of lay people's abilities in self-management, are recognised as potential obstacles. In response, recommendations are made to improve training of doctors, nurses and other healthcare professionals, and include the patient's voice more clearly within health care provision.

Greater inclusion of patients within healthcare was seen to be possible through: including and promoting users as active in their care; enabling patients to have informed choice; making health services responsive to the needs of users; ensuring users have skills and knowledge to influence NHS policies and planning through producing and disseminating information; resourcing organisational and structural changes; supporting staff, research and evaluation at national and local levels.

Some of the concerns anticipated in this government document have been articulated. For example, Shaw and Baker (2004) explain how doctors, already coping with patients who are increasingly armed with potentially dubious internet information, fear being overwhelmed by 'overbearing, too knowledgeable patients', and that developing patient partnerships will prove time consuming and costly. However, they point out that existing social inequalities mean that the majority of those with chronic conditions will lack the education and resources necessary to challenge their doctor's opinion. Nevertheless, Shaw and Baker (2004) feel that issues of responsibility and skill recognition within such partnership building could be more sensitively implemented and suggest that rather than refer to patients as experts, 'involved patents' would indicate a more egalitarian relationship.

It is felt that current undergraduate training of doctors still needs to focus more on chronic conditions and Garden (2005) suggest curriculums should include greater utilisation of community resources and the softer sciences of sociology and psychology. However, they recognise that this may prove less attractive to medical students and be unwelcome to current educators who may consider such changes as 'dumbing down'. Personal experience as a psychologist working with health educators has indeed meant hearing such concerns articulated. Nevertheless, there is increasing involvement of patients in training health professionals. For example, Allahlafi and Burge (2007) suggest that patient involvement in relation to chronic conditions such as psoriasis is vital to enable medical students to be aware of the emotional impact of such illness.

Nurses have also been found to be particularly uncomfortable with new initiatives such as the EPP, feeling vulnerable to litigation and reduced responsibility. However, Wilson et al. (2006) see a need for changes within nurse education and culture to help allay such fears.

Greater involvement of patient and user representatives now exists at many levels within healthcare training, including patients' involvement as teachers and in curriculum design and validation. However, there would appear to still be some way to go, as some patients still report that their doctors do not ask their opinion, set goals, or discuss emotional demands or how to cope, but are more comfortable when dealing with straightforward medical issues (Cooper 2007). Through their systematic review of patient involvement, Crawford et al. (2002) found that, despite increased evidence of patient participation within health services, there was no real indication of any improvements in terms of patients' health, quality of care or sense of satisfaction.

Smith (2002) suggests that there will always be limits on how far patients' views can be acted upon within healthcare. He recognises a tension between individuals' choices and the needs of their whole social group, and points out that healthcare professionals have constantly to balance often opposing needs. He refers to the public response to publication of conflicting concerns in relation to the MMR vaccine, prostate cancer screening and use of mammograms. Decisions made regarding such complex issues are difficult, even for the most informed professionals. Nevertheless, Smith (2002) cites some progress in the inclusion of patients' voices within healthcare given that patient representatives were included in a recent working party set up by Chief Medical Officer regarding chronic fatigue. However, that half of those in the working party had resigned before the report was published, and patients' views were dismissed by some medical experts as anecdotal suggests that there is still much more to be done to ensure patient involvement is valued.

Whilst there may be a need for greater sensitivity in how new patient–professional partnerships are implemented, and evaluation of their success, some important changes in both thinking and practice have been made within current healthcare. This reflects an increasing move towards adopting a bio-psycho-social view of patients, and particularly those with chronic conditions. As pointed out by Taylor and Bury (2007), and demonstrated through reference at the start of this chapter to Bronfenbrenner's bio-ecological theory, recognising the social and emotional impact of chronic illness is a means of meeting individuals' needs, as their health cannot be seen in isolation from their social context.

Conclusion

An attempt has been made within this chapter to:

- Demonstrate the impossibility of separating biological, psychological and social factors when considering patients' experiences of chronic illness. The raw material from which people develop is essentially biological and comprised of genetically inherited characteristics, but such development is shaped by social circumstances and involves experiencing psychological states.
- Illustrate how social inequalities, in terms of the social groups to which a person belongs, including class, gender and ethnicity, can impact upon health. This can be in terms of levels of control and linked to the opportunity for variety and choice over work and lifestyle, and can be felt as stressful.
- Examine current biological and cognitive explanations of stress. Information based on psychoneuroimmunology and cognitive theories was offered to explain how stress impacts on, and may be exacerbated by, chronic illness.
- Explore intervention strategies helpful when living with chronic conditions. National initiatives, such as the EPP and philosophy of patient partnerships were considered, but caution expressed, as these require a considerable change of thinking by both patients and health professionals. Despite a need for further evaluation, such increased mutual respect was seen as a move in the right direction for helping to cope with chronic conditions.

References

Abramson L.Y., Seligman M.E.P. and Teasdale J.D. (1978) Learned helplessness in humans: critique and reformulation. *Journal of Abnormal Psychology* 87(1): 49–74.

Acheson D. (1998) Independent inquiry into inequalities in health. In G. Davey Smith, D. Dorling and M. Shaw (eds) (2001) *Poverty, Inequality and Health in Britain, 1800–2000: A reader*. Bristol: Policy Press.

Allahlafi A. and Burge S. (2007) What should undergraduate medical students know about psoriasis? Involving patients in curriculum development: modified Delphi technique. *British Medical Journal*. 330: 633–636.

Apter M. (1997) Reversal theory: what is it? *The Psychologist* 10: 217–220.

Bandura A. (1977) Self-efficacy: Toward a unifying theory of behavioral change. *Psychological Review* 8(2): 191–215.

Barlow J.H., Turner A.P. and Wright C.C. (2000) A randomized controlled study of the Arthritis Self Management Programme in the UK. *Health Education Research* 15: 665–80.

Barlow J.H., Ellard D.R., Hainsworth J.M., Jones F.R. and Fisher A. (2005) A review of self-management interventions for panic disorders, phobias and obsessive-compulsive disorders. *Acta Psychiatrica Scandinavica* 111: 272–85.

Battersby M. (2006) A risk worth taking. *Chronic Illness* 2: 265–9.

Bennett P. and Murphy S. (2001) *Psychology and Health Promotion.* Buckingham: Open University Press.

Bosna H., Dike van de Mheen J. and Mackenbach J.P. (1999) Social class in childhood and general health in adulthood: questionnaire study of contribution of psychological attributes. *British Medical Journal* 318: 18–22.

Bronfenbrenner U. (1979) *The Ecology of Human Development: Experiments by the nature and design.* Cambridge, Mass: Harvard University Press.

Bronfenbrenner U. (2005) *Making Human Beings Human: Bioecological perspectives on human development.* Thousand Oaks, CA. Sage Publications.

Brooker S., Morris M. and Johnson A. (2008) Empowered to change: evidence from a qualitative exploration of a user informed psycho-educational programme for people with type 1 diabetes. *Chronic Illness* 4: 41–53.

Bury M. (2001) Illness narratives: fact or fiction? *Sociology of Health and Illness* 23(3): 263–85.

Bury M. (2004) Researching patient–professional interactions. *Journal of Health Services Research and Policy* 9(Suppl 1): S48–S54.

Buszewickz M., Rait G., Griffin M., Nazareth I., Patel A., Atkinson A., Barlow J. and Haines A. (2006) Self-management of arthritis in primary care: randomized controlled trial. *British Medical Journal* doi:10.1136/bmj.38965.37577188.80 (accessed 9 July 2007).

Campo J.V., Bridge J., Ehmann M., Altman S., Juca A., Birmaher B., DiLorenzo C., Iyengar S. and Brent D. (2004) Recurrent abdominal pain, anxiety, and depression in primary care. *Pediatrics* 13: 817–24.

Cannon W.B. (1929) *Bodily Changes in Pain, Hunger, Fear and Rage*, 2nd edn. New York: Norton.

Castes M., Hagal I., Palenque M., Corao A. and Lynch N.R. (1999) Immunological changes associated with clinical improvement of asthmatic children subjected to psychosocial intervention. *Brain, Behavior and Immunity* 13: 1–13.

Cooper J. (2007) *The Expert Patient.* Self-Management, Long-Term Conditions Alliance (LMCA). http://www.digg.org.uk/expert%20patient/expert3.asp (accessed 9 July 2007).

Crawford M.J., Rutter D., Manley C., Weaver T., Bindi K., Fulop N. and Tyrer P. (2002) Systematic review of involving patients in the planning and development of health care. *British Medical Journal* 325: 1263–7.

Danoff-Burg S., Agee J.D., Romanoff N.R., Kremer J.M. and Strosberg J.M. (2006) Benefit finding and expressive writing in adults with lupus or rheumatoid arthritis. *Psychology and Health* 21(5): 651–65.

Davey Smith G., Dorling D. and Shaw M. (eds) (2001) *Poverty, Inequality and Health in Britain, 1800–2000: a reader*. Bristol: Policy Press.

Davidson K., Gidron Y., Mostofsky E. and Trudeau K.J. (2007) Hospitalization cost offset of a hostility intervention for coronary heart disease patients. *Journal of Consulting and Clinical Psychology* 75(4): 657–662.

Dekkers J.C., Geenen R., Evers A.W.M., Kraaimaat F.W., Bijlsma J.W.J. and Godaert G.L.R. (2001) Biopsychosocial mediators and moderators of stress-health relationships in patients with recently diagnosed rheumatoid arthritis. *Arthritis Care and Research* 45: 307–16.

Department of Health (DH) (1997) *Patient partnership: Building a Collaborative Strategy*. London: The Stationery Office.

Department of Health (DH) (2000) *The Expert Patient: A new Approach to Chronic Disease Management for the 21st Century*. London: The Stationery Office.

Dixon K., Keefe F.J., Scipio C.D., Perri L.M. and Abernethy A.P. (2007) Psychological interventions for arthritis pain management in adults: a meta-analysis. *Health Psychology* 26: 241–50.

Donaldson L. (2003) Expert patients usher in a new era of opportunity for the NHS. *British Medical Journal* 326: 1279.

Evans P., Clow A. and Hucklebridge F. (1997) Stress and the immune system. *The Psychologist* 10: 303–7.

Evers A.W., Lu Y., Duller P., van der Valk P.G., Kraaimaat F.W. and van de Kerkhof P.C. (2005) Common burden of chronic skin diseases? Contributors to psychological distress in adults with psoriasis and atopic dermatitis. *British Journal of Dermatology* 152(6): 1275–81.

Feder G., Crook A.M., Magee P., Banerjee S., Timmis A.D. and Hemingway H. (2002) Ethnic differences in invasive management of coronary disease: prospective cohort study of patients undergoing angiography. *British Medical Journal* 324: 511–16.

Ferguson E., Matthews G. and Cox T. (1999) Appraisal of Life Events (A.L.E.) Scale. Reliability and Validity. *British Journal of Health Psychology* 4: 97–116.

Field D. and Payne S. (2003) Social aspects of bereavement. *Cancer Nursing Practice* 2(8): 21–5.

Finn L. (2006) Pluralistic responses to the challenge of chronic illness. *Chronic Illness* 2: 270–1.

Folkman S., Lazarus R.S., Gruen R.J. and DeLongis A. (1986) Appraisal, coping, health statues and psychological symptoms. *Journal of Personality and Social Psychology* 50: 571–9.

Frankenhaeuser M. (1980) Psychological aspects of life stress. In S. Levine and H. Ursin (eds) *Coping and Health*. New York: Plenum.

Garden A. (2005) Chronic disease: the challenge for medical education. *Chronic Illness* 1: 277.

Griffiths C., Foster G., Ramsay J., Eldridge S. and Taylor S. (2007) How effective are expert patient (lay led) education programmes for chronic disease? *British Medical Journal* 334: 1254–6.

Grundy E. and Glaser K. (2000) Socio-demographic differences in the onset and progression of disability in early old age: a longitudinal study. *Age and Ageing* 29: 149–57.

Halligan P. (2007) Belief and illness. *The Psychologist* 20(6): 358–61.

Hamilton-West K.E. and Quine L. (2007) Effects of written emotional disclosure on health outcomes in patients with ankylosing spondylitis. *Psychology and Health* 22(6): 637–57.

Hawton K., Salkovskis P.M., Kirk J. and Clark D.M. (1989) *Cognitive Behaviour Therapy for Psychiatric Problems*. Oxford: Oxford Medical Publications.

Hennessy M.B., Deak T. and Schiml-Webb P.A. (2001) Stress-induced sickness behaviors: an alternative hypothesis for responses during maternal separation. *Developmental Psychobiology* 39: 76–83.

Hippisley-Cox J., Fielding K. and Pringle M. (1998) Depression as a risk factor for ischaemic heart disease in men: population based case-control study. *British Medical Journal* 316: 1714–9.

Holman H.R. (2005) Chronic disease and the healthcare crisis. *Chronic Illness* 1: 265–74.

Holman H.R. (2007) What should be incentivized in care of chronic illness? *Chronic Illness* 3: 194–5.

Holman H.R. and Lorig K.R. (1997) Patient education: essential to good health care for patients with chronic arthritis. *Arthritis and Rheumatism* 40(8): 1371–3.

Kiecolt-Glaser J.K. (1999) Stress, personal relationships, and immune function: health implications. *Brain, Behaviour and Immunity* 13: 61–72.

Kiviruusu O., Huurre T. and Aro H. (2007) Psychosocial resources and depression among chronically ill young adults: Are males more vulnerable? *Social Science and Medicine* 65(2): 173–86.

Kovacs M. (2007) Stress and coping in the workplace. *The Psychologist* 20(9): 548–50.

Kuijer R.G., De Ridder D.T.D., Colland V.T., Schreurs K.M.G. and Spraners M.A.G. (2007) Effects of a short self-management intervention for patients with asthma and diabetes: Evaluating health-related quality of life using then-test methodology. *Psychology and Health* 22(4): 387–411.

Lau-Walker M. (2006) Predicting self-efficacy using illness perception components: a patient survey. *British Journal of Health Psychology* 11: 643–61.

Lazarus R.S. and Folkman S. (1984) *Stress Appraisal and Coping*. New York: Springer.

Lemert E.M. (1972) *Human Deviance, Social Problems, and Social Control*, 2nd edn. Engelwood Cliffs: Prentice-Hall.

Lynch J.W., Davey Smith G., Kaplan G.A. and House J.S. (2000) Income inequality and morality: importance to health of individual income, psychosocial environment, or material conditions. *British Medical Journal* 320: 1200–4.

Lowe R., Cockshott Z., Greenwood R., Krwan J.R., Almeida C., Richards P. and Hewlett S. (2007) Self-efficacy as an appraisal that moderates the coping-emotion relationship: associations among people with rheumatoid arthritis. *Psychology and Health* 23(2): 155–74.

Lucas T., Alexander S., Firestone I. and Lebreton J.M. (in press) Just world beliefs, perceived stress, and health behaviour: the impact of a procedurally just world. *Psychology and Health* 10.1080/08870440701456020.

Maiden N., Capell J.A., Madhok R., Hampson R. and Thompson E.A. (1999) Does social disadvantage contribute to the excess mortality in RA patients? *Annals of Rheumatic Diseases* 58: 525–9.

Marmot M. and Wilkinson R.G. (2001) Psychosocial and material pathways in the elation between income and health: a response to Lynch et al. *British Medical Journal* 322: 1233–6.

Marmot M.G., Shipley M.J. and Rose G. (1984) Inequalities in death – specific explanations of a general pattern? *Lancet* I(5): 1003–6.

Marmot M.G., Smith D. and Stansfield S.A. (1991) Health inequalities among British civil servants: the Whitehall Study II. *Lancet* 337: 1387–93.

Moos R.H. and Holahan C.J. (2003) Dispositional and contextual perspectives on coping: toward an integrative framework. *Journal of Clinical Psychology* 59(12): 1387–403.

Nelson-Jones R. (2001) *Theory and Practice of Counselling Therapy.* London: Continuum.

Nettleton S. (2000) *The Sociology of Health and Illness.* London: Polity Press.

Newbould J., Taylor D. and Bury M. (2006) Lay-led self-management in chronic illness: a review of the evidence. *Chronic Illness* 2: 249–61.

Ockleford E., Shaw R.L., Willars J. and Dixon-Woods M. (2008) Education and self-management for people newly diagnosed with type 2 diabetes: a qualitative study of patients' views. *Chronic Illness* 4: 28–37.

O'Donovan A. and Hughes B.M. (2006) Your best interest at heart? *The Psychologist* 19(4): 216–19.

Peckham S. and Meerabeau L. (2007) *Social Policy for Nurses and the Helping Professionals*, 2nd edn. Maidenhead: Open University Press.

Phillips A.C. and Burns V.E. (2008) A shot in the arm for research. *The Psychologist* 21(3): 202–4.

Plach S.K. (2008) Psychological well-being in women with heart failure: can social-roles make a difference? *Health Care for Women International* 29: 54–75.

Porter M., Abraham B. and Alder C. (1999) *Psychology and Sociology Applied to Medicine.* London: Churchill Livingstone.

Rhee S.H., Parker J.C., Smarr K.L., Petroski G.F., Johnson J.C., Hewett J.E. et al. (2000) Stress management in rheumatoid arthritis: What is the underlying mechanism? *Arthritis Care and Research* 13: 435–42.

Rhodes P.J., Small N.A., Ismail H. and Wright J.P. (2008) 'What really annoys me is people take it like it's a disability', epilepsy, disability and identity among people of Pakistani origin living in the UK. *Ethnicity and Health* 13(1): 1–21.

Rogers A. (2006) Damned by faint praise. *Chronic Illness* 2: 263–4.

Rotter J.B. (1966) Generalised expectations for internal versus external control of reinforcement. *Psychological Monographs* 80.

Ryan S., Hassell A.B., Dawes P.T. and Kendall S. (2003) Control perceptions in patients with rheumatoid arthritis: the role of social support. *Musculoskeletal Care* 1(2): 108–18.

Sapey B. (2001) From stigma to the social exclusion of disabled people. In T. Mason, C. Carlisle, C. Watkins and E. Whitehead (eds) *Stigma and Social Exclusion in Healthcare*. London: Routledge, pp. 270–9.

Sareen J., Cox B.J., Clara I. and Asmundson G.J.G. (2005) The relationship between anxiety disorders and physical disorders in the U.S. National comorbidity survey. *Depression and Anxiety* 21: 193–202.

Seligman M.E. and Maier S.F. (1975) Failure to escape traumatic shock. *Journal of Experimental Psychology* 74(1): 1–9.

Selye H. (1956) *The Stress of Life*. New York: McGraw-Hill.

Senior V., Weinman J. and Marteau T.M. (2002) The influence of perceived oconrol over causes and responses to health threats: a vignette study. *British Journal of Health Psychology* 7: 203–11.

Shaw J. and Baker M. (2004) 'Expert patient' – dream or nightmare? *British Medical Journal* 328: 723–4.

Sheehy C., Murphy E. and Barry M. (2006) *Rheumatology* 45: 1325–7.

Sherman A.M., Shumaker S.A., Rejeski W.J., Morgan T., Applegate W.B. and Ettinger W. (2006) *Psychology and Health* 21(4): 463–80.

Smith J.A. and Osborn M. (2007) Pain as an assault on the self: an interpretative phenomenological analysis of the psychological impact of chronic benign low back pain. *Psychology and Health* 22(5): 517–34.

Smith R. (2002) The discomfort of patient power. *British Medical Journal* 324: 497–8.

Smyth M.M., Stone A.A., Hurwitz A. and Kaell A. (1999) Effects of writing about stressful experiences on symptoms reduction in patients with asthma or rheumatoid arthritis, a randomized trial. *Journal of the American Medical Association* 281: 1304–9.

Stowell J.R., Kiecolt-Glaser J.K. and Glaser R. (2001) Perceived stress and cellular immunity: When coping counts. *Journal of Behavioral Medicine* 24(4): 323–9.

Straub R.H., Shabha F.S., Bijlsa W.J. and Cutolo M. (2005) How psychological stress via hormones and nerve fibers may exacerbate rheumatoid arthritis. *Arthritis and Rheumatism* 52(1): 16–26.

Taylor D. and Bury M. (2007) Chronic illness, expert patients and care transition. *Sociology of Health and Illness* 29(1): 27–45.

Thomas A. and Chess S. (1977) *Temperament and Development*. New York: Bremner Mazel.

Thomas B. and Dorling D. (2007) *Identity in Britain: A Cradle-to-grave Atlas.* Bristol. Bristol: Policy Press.

Thompson A.R., Kent G. and Smith J.A. (2002) Living with vitiligo: dealing with difference. *British Journal of Health Psychology.* 7: 213–25.

Townend P., Davidson N. and Whitehead M. (1992) *Inequalities in Health: The Black Report; The Health Divide.* Hammondsworth: Penguin.

Treharne G.J., Lyons A.C., Booth D.A. and Kitas G.D. (2007) Psychological well-being across 1 year with rheumatoid arthritis: Coping resources as buffers of perceived stress. *British Journal of Health Psychology* 12: 323–45.

Trilling J.S. (2000) Psychoneuroimmunology: validation of the biopsychosocial model. *Family Practice* 17: 90–3.

Vandyke M.M., Parker J.C., Smarr K.L., Hewett J.E., Johnson G.E., Slaughter J.R. and Walker S.E. (2004) Anxiety in rheumatoid arthritis. *Arthritis and Rheumatism* 51(3): 408–12.

Vargas L.E., Pena P.M.L. and Vargas M.A. (2006) Influence of anxiety in diverse cutaneous diseases. *Actas Dermosifiliographicas* 97(10): 637–43.

Waite-Jones J.M. (1998) Stress and Rheumatoid Arthritis: A Qualitative Approach. University of Manchester: unpublished MSc thesis.

Waite-Jones J.M. (2005) Juvenile Idiopathic Arthritis and Family Function. University of Leeds: unpublished PhD thesis.

Wilson P.M., Kendall S. and Brooks F. (2006) Nurses' responses to expert patients: the rhetoric and reality of self-management in long-term conditions: A grounded theory study. *International Journal of Nursing Studies* 43: 803–18.

Younger J., Finan P., Zautra A., Davis M. and Reich J. (2008) Personal mastery predicts pain, stress, fatigue, and blood pressure in adults with rheumatoid arthritis. *Psychology and Health* 23(5): 515–35.

Chapter 4

Pain psychology

Joan Maclean

Introduction

The aim of this chapter is to distil some useful points from the vast amount of pain literature students will find when seeking information about the psychology of pain. How do pain theories link with the behaviours which may be observed out in practice? What psychological concepts can really help us understand individual responses to pain, and have they been drawn upon in clinical environments? Psychosocial variables such as sex and culture are explored for their impact upon pain responses, and the extent to which this can help in practice is discussed. Finally, brief reference is made to interventions with a psychological basis which may augment pharmacological approaches to pain management.

It is beyond the scope of this chapter to explore in any depth specialist psychological assessment in pain management. Rather, its content should help the student to apply some straightforward psychological concepts – which may indeed have been studied at an introductory level – to the experience and expression of pain in their own patient or client group. Similarly, methods of pain measurement and the range of approaches employed are not discussed in detail here, although measurement will arise in the context of specific studies. Experimental measurement of pain usually involves assessment of sensitivity and tolerance; methods of producing short-term pain for empirical studies may include thermal techniques such as heat producing electrodes, or cold pressor tests involving immersion of a digit or limb. Other methods include electric shock or application of irritants. In the reality of a clinical setting these may be of less use, and more subjective reporting methods by way of verbal rating or visual analogue may be more valuable. For more detailed reading about pain measurement and management the student could look at Horn and Munafo (1997), Schofield (2005), or Main et al. (2008).

Pain definitions offer varying combinations of these fundamental points: pain is unpleasant, comprises sensory and affective factors, and is frequently but not unfailingly an indication of injured or impaired tissue. Acute pain produces a characteristic autonomic response – an increase in respiration, heart rate and arterial pressure, accompanied by palmar sweating, pupillary dilation and increased muscle tension. Its disturbing quality is summarised more prosaically by the protagonist Winston Smith in Orwell's dystopian classic novel (1949): 'Of pain you could wish only one thing: that it should stop.'

What is clear from the wealth of literature, and becomes even clearer as clinical experience develops, is the number of facets to the pain experience, including physiological, behavioural, emotional and socio-cultural factors. Though an understanding of the variety of factors is undoubtedly of help to healthcare practitioners, it is important to remember that the individual actually suffering the pain may need a more gentle introduction to the notion of anything other than an organic or physiological element to their pain. Main et al. (2008) note the potential for some patients referred for psychological assessment in the course of chronic pain management to adopt a negative view of psychology as a tool, perhaps seeing this as a step towards demonstrating that their pain is all in their mind, or that there is some mental health problem. Yet we can see the place for a psychological understanding even as we study the physiology of pain. Pain is distracting, it is intrusive, and it hurts. The majority of us do not wish to hurt, hence the very natural desire to avoid and remove pain, and the generation of strong emotions – distress, anxiety, anger – in response to the experience.

Acute pain has a warning function: it alerts us to the possibility that something may be wrong. It follows therefore that the thankfully rare anomaly of congenital insensitivity to pain – congenital analgesia – must be a burdensome rather than a happy condition. The absence of any functional warning system means a reduced ability to note injury, and, more important according to Wall (2000), no real urge to protect an injured area thereby allowing recovery. The ensuing accumulation of unrepaired tissue may lead to chronic damage and possible life-threatening complications.

Where acute pain is time-limited (although there are differing opinions as to this limit), chronic pain may occur when pain is experienced over a prolonged period. The pain may be subsequent to an initial acute event, or as a result of some long-term condition, for example rheumatoid arthritis or cancer, or on occasion there may be no apparent root cause. Chronic pain has a tendency to disrupt activity and detract from quality of life, and is a challenge to its sufferers, their families, and the practitioners who seek to relieve it. We see the warning or survival aspect of acute pain, yet it is difficult to discern a purpose for chronic pain, unless perhaps religious beliefs lead one to any conclusion regarding its strengthening of any spiritual state.

If it is hard for the practitioner to understand and articulate this, how much more demanding must it be of the individual in pain? The patient may have experience of both types of pain with the same root cause: an episode of acute pain brought about by trauma may be followed by longstanding complex pain disorder; likewise the person with cancer may endure acute pain associated with surgery, which is later followed by chronic pain associated with a number of circumstances including chemotherapy, radiotherapy and possibly the development of metastases. What becomes apparent when one explores chronic or longstanding pain is that this understanding must be expanded in order to appreciate what is happening to the patient. Persistent or chronic pain may be associated with different processes. Barash et al. (2006) note that nociceptors may have altered sensitivity, substances which modulate pain may act differently, and the action of analgesic drugs such as opiates may be modified. In addition, psychological and emotional factors continue to have an effect, meaning that a holistic assessment of the patient is indicated, where psychology is explored alongside physical and pathological processes. A range of psychological effects may accompany chronic pain, including sleep disturbances, fatigue and outright exhaustion, sadness, anger and irritability. None of these is surprising in the face of relentless pain, and no huge leap of thinking is required to realise that depression may arise in the chronic pain sufferer, although the order of onset may be harder to unravel. Does chronic pain beget depression, is the depressed person more susceptible to experiencing chronic pain, or is it some combination of the two? A more detailed and critical discussion of acute versus chronic pain is available in Horn and Munafo (1997).

Pain physiology and pain theory

Pain occurs in response to noxious stimulation which triggers the release of algogenic or pain-producing chemicals – for example histamine, bradykinin, serotonin – at the site of injury or damage (Chapman 1984). These activate nociceptors, which are free nerve endings found throughout body tissue. The afferent neurons enter the spinal cord via the dorsal roots, and synapse in the dorsal horns with the secondary neurons. These neurons, components of the lateral spinothalamic tract, travel up through the brain stem to the thalamus. Their routes include the epicritic pathway – small myelinated A-delta fibres which transmit sharp, bright pain at around 5–30 m/sec and serve skin and mucous membranes, and the protopathic pathway – very small unmyelinated C fibres which transmit dull, throbbing pain at around 0.5–2 m/sec and serve all skin and body tissue except insensitive brain tissue (Tortora and Anagnostakis 1990). Some awareness may occur at thalamic, therefore sub-cortical, level; other impulses will pass through to the sensory and motor areas of the cortex allowing recognition of their source and severity.

Pain physiology, then, describes the workings of pain pathways, and allows us to see what is happening physically to the individual; alongside this sits a collection of *pain theories* which offer a framework for our evolved understanding of the concept of pain. Descartes proposed a 'straight through' transmission of pain, referred to as the 'bell pull' analogy since it described a signal which travelled from the area of stimulus up the spinal cord to the brain, thereby resulting in sensation. The mechanism was thus separate from the experience, with little apparent notion of any psychological component. Much later this Cartesian notion was expanded by Von Frey's theory of specificity (1894), which added detail to the concept but remained quite mechanistic. It described four skin-based senses or modalities – touch, warmth, cold and pain – each with its own projection, or specific pathway, to a responsible area of the brain. Von Frey's ideas underpinned much 20th-century research into the pathways, transmission and localisation of pain.

An alternative model which became known as the pattern theory – described by Goldscheider (1894) – refuted the notions of either straight-through transmission or Von Frey's ideas of specificity, suggesting instead that pain arose from synchronised impulses from the stimulated area impinging at once on the cortex, via the spinal cord. Summation of stimuli at the dorsal horn – the amount and spacing of input – was deemed to be the significant factor influencing pain, although this would not explain the phenomenon of slight stimulation leading to severe pain – for example in trigeminal or post-herpetic neuralgias. However, elements of this pattern theory influenced the development of the more complex and dynamic *gate control theory* (Melzack and Wall 1965). The 'gate' in question is a hypothetical mechanism at spinal cord level which is assumed to modulate peripheral nerve signals before they reach the cortex – so before perception is evoked – by influencing the flow of impulses. The gate setting depends upon a balance of activity which includes:

- the amount of activity in A-delta (epicritic) and C (protopathic) pain fibres
- the amount of activity in other peripheral fibres, in particular large diameter A-beta fibres carrying irritation information
- descending messages from brain – that is, centrally initiated impulses.

The one-directional notion put forward by Descartes is therefore somewhat undone by the gate control theory, which proposes that modulation can arise both centrally and peripherally. The influence of central activity means that emotional states have the potential to impact upon pain perception, and thus an individual's apparent pain level, or experience, may appear disproportionate to injury. As the late Patrick Wall, whose writing on pain is some of the most accessible and useful students can read, observed: 'Public display of pain and the expression of suffering are full of surprises. The amount of pain and the amount of injury are not tightly coupled (Wall 2000)'.

A classic illustration of this phenomenon, and one which fuelled experts' interest and underpinned such theoretical developments, is Beecher's study of pain perception in military casualties in the Second World War. Beecher noted that pain levels appeared inconsistent with the extent of wounds, and on admission to hospital it was observed that men were declining analgesia and denying injury-related pain, despite being seriously wounded. This paradox was explained in terms of euphoria at removal from the site of battle; indeed Beecher described an apparently exalted state in some soldiers. Yet in civilians with proportionate injury sustained in non-military circumstances, pain report and relief required appeared to be greater (Beecher 1956).

Beecher's 'episodic analgesia' and gate control theory, then, suggest to us that pain may be modulated by descending activity as well as by the impinging stimulus. But does emotion inhibit or amplify the pain experience? Rhudy and Meagher (2001) discuss the interaction between valence and arousal, where valence is a measure of pleasantness versus unpleasantness, and arousal a measure of calmness versus excitability. Using sets of visual stimuli and a cold pressor test, their findings indicated that negative emotion with only moderate arousal may amplify pain, while positive emotion reduces it. However, highly arousing negative emotion – for example in a situation where fear is a factor – may in fact inhibit pain.

Can we link this with stress response? We have seen that stress, like pain, is a highly adaptive response as previously mentioned in Chapter 3, and it may be that a temporary dampening of pain perception is helpful in the face of danger. Add to this the mechanism of endogenous opioid release as a feature of the stress response, and we can see a picture emerging to support and add to Beecher's earlier accounts of episodic analgesia.

Drawing upon the premise of gate control, certain subsequent models have sought to explain further the emotional component of pain. A four-stage model by Wade et al. (1992), derived in part from work by Price (1988), presented four identifiable stages in the experience of pain (Figure 4.1):

1. pain sensation intensity – the sensory dimension
2. pain unpleasantness, an immediate affective response involving limited cognitive processes, and closely associated with sensation
3. long-term cognition, suffering, where implications of pain for the individual may lead to feelings of anxiety or fear, representing the psychological component, considered unique and therefore separate from stages 1 and 2
4. pain behaviour.

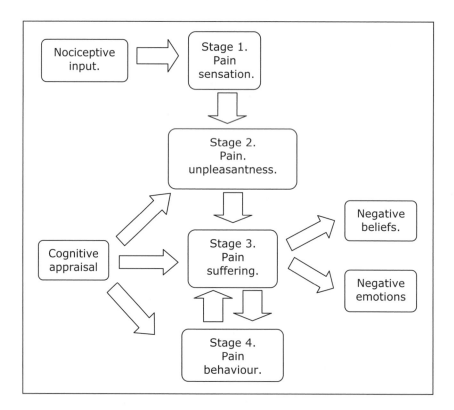

Figure 4.1 A four-stage model in the experience of pain. Source: Wade et al. (1988).

It may be helpful to superimpose such a model on a typically painful event to enhance comprehension of the patient's experience. For example, the pain of myocardial infarction, while naturally varying among individuals (and indeed, in a silent infarction, pain may not be a symptom at all) is often described as severe, located in the chest, with possible radiation to the jaw and the arms, in particular the left arm. However, chest pain and nausea can also be symptoms of dyspepsia. Stages 1 and 2 of Wade's model would pick up the sensory and deeply unpleasant nature of this chest pain. Stage 3, which encompasses implications, may differentiate between those who would consider chest pain as cardiac related and therefore potentially life threatening, and those without such expectations who might initially assume nothing more than an attack of indigestion and heartburn. So while stage 4, pain behaviour, may find both individuals nauseated and shocked because of the sensory pain, attributions and associated anxiety and fear may present quite differently.

Such models support the concept of pain as a personal experience but also may allow us to interpret pain as it is presented in a practice situation. These suggestions regarding the part played by emotion may help us to 'read' the situation when trying to manage pain. In what context is the pain stimulus occurring? What might the patient be feeling and thinking, and how negative or threatening are those thoughts? Price (1999) has noted that we may all be disposed to perceive pain as an unpleasant thing since it so often accompanies a threatening event. It is certainly a very frequent and common symptom of an illness, which is in itself a potential threat, or it may occur in the event of a traumatic accident, punishment or a physical fight, all of which may be considered negative experiences.

Expectation and motivation

Certain psychological variables may have a moderating influence on the affective or emotional aspect of pain. Price et al. (1980) demonstrated this in a study where participants were subjected to pain induced via thermal skin stimuli. If a warning signal was given prior to the stimulus, then the unpleasantness of the pain (that is, the affective component) was judged to be reduced, despite the pain sensation (that is, the sensory component) remaining similar to that in the no warning state. In the laboratory setting then, this would indicate that receiving warning of imminent pain may temper the unpleasantness of the experience if not the actual sensation.

Studies such as this offer findings which are extremely useful to the assessment and care of the patient in pain. If we move away from pain experienced in this dislocated manner in a laboratory setting, we can see how these ideas might translate into practice. Most health professionals study, early on in their programmes of education, the importance of communication skills, in relation to both receiving and conveying information. We are encouraged to let people know what has happened, what is happening and what will happen to them (to the extent that we can predict this). Expectations in relation to pain, therefore, may be managed in some way by communicating with the patient to let them know what is to happen, allowing them the courtesy of prediction – to tell them that this procedure is likely to be painful, but we will try not to let it take them by surprise.

Pain can arise from any number of sources, and – as pain measurement techniques show – it can vary quantitatively and qualitatively both in the same individual across time, and among individuals undergoing similar experiences. The notions of expectation and motivation can help us understand the responses to pain across different situations. For example, the affective response to pain associated with cancer may differ from that experienced in labour, or as a result of elective cosmetic surgery. Price et al. (1987) undertook a comparison of groups experiencing clinical pain, including chronic pain, labour and birth, cancer pain and experimental pain; the findings demonstrated this potential for motivation to influence pain perception. Measuring both the sensory and the affective aspect of pain allowed evidence of this difference to emerge: the cancer patients rated the unpleasantness aspect of their pain more highly than the sensory aspect, while for the women in labour the sensory ratings were greater than those of unpleasantness. It may be then that variance in expectations and connotations of pain may have an influence on perception of pain. The implication of pain in a person with cancer – advances in treatment notwithstanding – may be one of threat and potential deterioration. In contrast the pain associated with labour and birth, though severe, could be said to imply a clear purpose and denote generation rather than limitation of life. This offers a slightly different take on the notion that somehow the emotional fulfilment of childbirth tempers the perception of labour pain for women, and indeed Salmon (1990) has demonstrated fulfilment, pain and unpleasantness to be independent factors in women in labour. Rather, it suggests that the pain of labour and delivery are strong and sensed, but it is the affective aspect which is tempered by the motivation and emotions involved.

One more physiological mechanism which may add to an understanding of pain is the release of endogenous opioids. These analgesic substances develop naturally within the body yet behave like opiates – that is, their action resembles that of drugs such as morphine which is derived from the opium poppy. The discovery of their existence and consequently their properties is relatively recent. The isolation of these substances, and discovery of an opiate receptor system within the central nervous system, occurred in the latter half of the 20th century (Snyder et al. 1974; Hughes et al. 1975). Released in sudden stress or injury, endogenous opioids are thought to react at receptor sites, reducing pain sensation. They contribute to descending signals closing the hypothetical gate in gate control, thereby possibly helping to bring about episodic analgesia such as that described by Beecher.

Pain behaviour

Pain may be universally recognised as a concept, yet its experience is inherently personal. Much as we would wish, we cannot 'take the pain' for a child or a loved relative who is suffering, nor can we fully experience it although we may feel familiarity with what is happening. How then can we surmise that someone is experiencing pain? One way is by recognising their behaviour. Given the importance of pain as a symptom, the ability to recognise pain behaviour in its wide-ranging form is a most important skill. Pain behaviour may include:

- facial expression – grimacing, screwing up eyes
- audible complaint – verbal or sub-verbal
- altered posture or gait – limping or rigidity
- reduced mobility
- guarded, exaggeratedly careful movement
- negative affect, low mood.

So in practice recognition of pain may come about by observing a patient or client grimacing, weeping, limping, protecting a body part, sitting very still, looking downcast, responding with irritation to people around him or her – or a mixture of all these things.

To try to understand this observed behaviour we can consider some behaviourist concepts, which can be most illuminating in the examination of health and illness behaviour, and especially so when considering pain. Pavlovian or *classical conditioning* occurs when a neutral stimulus is paired with an unconditioned stimulus, resulting in the unconditioned or reflex response becoming conditioned. Pavlov demonstrated this by conditioning a salivation response in dogs to a previously neutral light/bell (Pavlov 1927). Morrow and Dobkin (1988) demonstrated a classically conditioned nausea response in patients

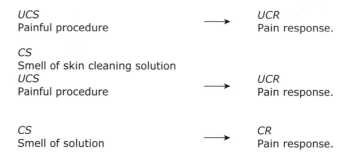

Figure 4.2 Classical conditioning and pain.

undergoing chemotherapy. The physiological events which accompany acute pain – tachycardia, sweating – may themselves be elicited by a conditioned stimulus in this way. For example, a particularly painful procedure carried out for the first time may be accompanied by a variety of neutral visual, auditory or even olfactory stimuli. Let us take the last type: if the procedure has involved the use of a particularly pungent antiseptic, then the smell of that antiseptic can come to signal imminent pain – that is it may be a conditioned stimulus, eliciting a reflex response – tachycardia, hyperarousal – without any pain stimulus being applied at all. This is diagrammatically represented in Figure 4.2).

A further illustration of this application of classical conditioning to pain is offered by Osgood and Szyfelbein (1989) who describe the demonstrated fear response, in advance of the procedure, in children awaiting the dressing of burn injuries; environmental events or objects such as nurses' masks are suggested as the conditioned stimuli.

Where classical conditioning refers to reflex responses, *operant conditioning*, as described by Skinner (1953) is on the whole associated with voluntary response. The outcome with which a behaviour meets will affect the strengthening or weakening of that haviour, and the likelihood of its being repeated. Brena and Chapman (1985) described how learned behaviour acquired by way of reinforcement may result in a learned pain syndrome comprising:

- dramatised complaint
- disuse through diminished activity
- drug misuse
- dependency
- disability.

How then can pain behaviour be reinforced? What positive outcome could there be for the individual displaying pain behaviour? Positive reinforcement might include renewal of attention or affection, while negative reinforcement may be the avoidance of going to work, to school, or of undertaking a particular item of work. Secondary gain may therefore become a component: pain is accepted as a cause of suffering, yet reinforcement of pain behaviours, whether positive as in increased attention, or negative as in avoidance of work, becomes a benefit arising from the pain. Barash et al. (2006) note the possibility that somatisation disorders may be in part maintained by operant conditioning, where the patient has learned – by picking up on available reinforcement – that the manifestation of a bodily symptom may meet with more attention and support than that of an emotional complaint.

Fordyce (1976) emphasised the relationship between behaviour and pain, and applied Skinnerian principles to pain behaviour to show how the concept of operant conditioning might explain in part patterns of behaviour which develop in individuals suffering chronic pain. Fordyce suggested that pain behaviours such as altered gait, reduced mobility, verbal complaint and anxiety could meet with reinforcing responses which through both their strength and their regularity may strengthen the behaviour; indeed positive reinforcement may not only strengthen pain expression but also reduce pain tolerance. A further idea posited by Fordyce was the inadvisability of administering analgesia on a pro re nata (prn – 'as need arises') basis. Here the patient has to report or demonstrate pain to receive pain relief, thus reinforcing pain behaviour. In addition Fordyce suggested that this approach might allow pain to build to such a level that there is a negative reinforcement also at play. Remember that negative reinforcement results in a strengthening or repeating of a behaviour which, though not intrinsically rewarding, allows the avoidance of an unpleasant event. Linking analgesia administration to time, rather than to manifest behaviour, is one way to avoid this, and the alternative strategy of administering a regular maintenance dose of analgesia could reduce the conditioning effect. As Patterson (2005) notes over 30 years on, the significance and influence of Fordyce's ideas can still be seen.

It has been suggested that operant conditioning can be used, with care, as the basis for attempts to increase 'well' behaviours in the patient with chronic pain. Though this may take time and expert guidance (Waters et al. 2004) the impact of reinforcement may be used in an attempt to reshape behaviours. Family members can be guided to alter their own response to the person in pain – that is to reduce the attention and solicitous attitude normally elicited by the pain behaviour – and instead try to strengthen their reinforcement of, for example, increased mobility and participation in activities.

Bandura's classic study of the *social learning* of aggressive behaviour (Bandura et al. 1961) demonstrated both vicarious and latent learning. Not all learning is direct, and a behaviour may be absorbed from a role model and imitated, yet this might not occur immediately, so the behaviour may not be demonstrated until a later point in time. The learning of pain behaviour by this route may be no exception. Think of the little child at nursery school who hurts its arm, and, assisted by a solicitous friend, limps over to the teacher for comfort. Why the hobble when the injury occurred at arm level? Has the child watched how others behave when injured? At a later stage, the menarche, one may observe young girls displaying pain behaviour related to menstrual periods, and wonder if there is a group effect, or some socially learned attitude to dysmenorrhoea which has been absorbed from mothers or other female relatives and friends. At a less specific level, debate about male and female response to pain – which is discussed in a little more depth later in this chapter – will always have reference to socially learned responses and the part they may play in sex differentiation.

Social learning may be worth considering, then, in relation to both pain expression and an individual's approach to pain. It is interesting to set this against the part that operant conditioning may play in an individual's pain behaviour. Stoicism in the face of pain may have been role modelled and indeed reinforced in early life, where attention to pain was scant, and yet this learning could imaginably be disadvantageous when pain is suffered at a later stage and must be conveyed to those who can help– that is, to health professionals.

Pain and culture

The pain experience may also be mediated by ethno-cultural processes. Seminal work which demonstrated variation in pain response among several different groups was carried out by Mark Zborowski in the USA, in an initial study of groups in the early 1950s, which was followed by a more extensive cross-cultural study of the effects of culture on the human experience of pain (Zborowski 1952, 1969). Zborowski observed that patients from different ethnic backgrounds had different responses when exposed to similar painful events – for example patients from one ethnic group might be highly anxious for pain relief but satisfied once this was relieved, while those from another were also anxious for pain relief, yet remained uneasy and fearful of implications despite successful analgesia. Still others would become withdrawn and quiet while suffering their pain. Subsequent investigation of pain thresholds across ethnic groups demonstrated no statistically significant differences (Sternbach and Tursky 1965) implying that while physiological processes may be homogeneous, expression and pain report may possibly be influenced by ethno-cultural variables.

A much more recent US based study of cancer patients who were asked to rate their pain (Greenwald 1991) highlights the differentiation between the sensory and affective components of pain. While sensory differences were not detected, there was a statistically significant difference among ethnic groups on ratings of the affective component of their pain. Conversely, very recent work by Campbell et al. (2008) did demonstrate difference in the sensorimotor response to painful electrical stimulus, between African American and white non-Hispanic groups, with results which suggested a lower threshold in the former ethnic group – and yet qualitative ratings were not significantly different.

These are just a few of very many studies. Should it come as any surprise to well-informed, thinking practitioners if people from different ethnic groups do respond differently to pain? Diverse groups have diverse experiences, and environment and learning may well influence an individual's pain response, including their pain behaviour and the outward manifestations of their pain. It is these overt aspects, as noted earlier in this chapter, which supply the observer with the information that someone is experiencing pain. The variation across individuals will become apparent to any observant health practitioner; what one would wish to avoid is the trap of stereotyping patients in relation to pain response, with any subsequent effect on the management of their pain. A study in the USA by Davitz and Davitz (1981) demonstrated the influence ethnic group might have on nurses' inferences of patients' suffering, while Todd et al. (2000) observed different analgesic practice in relation to black and white patients who had sustained orthopaedic injury. Lasch (2000) has reviewed the literature relating to ethnocultural pain differences and argued that a culturally sensitive approach plays a most important part in effective pain management.

The presence of immigrant populations from an increasing number of regions has had a noticeable impact on healthcare. The shaping of perceptions and world view by culture and ethnicity does appear to extend to pain response, and an understanding of this enhances the approach to caring and pain management for all patient groups.

Pain and sex difference

Just as cultural or ethnic stereotypes may suggest difference in pain response, so may sex or gender have an influence. We must remember however that while sex is, strictly speaking, biologically determined, gender may be a different issue, incorporating notions of ascription. Thus the mix of physiological and psychological processes involved in pain must be borne in mind when considering any apparent sex difference in pain perception or response, and the question asked: could this have a physiological underpinning in addition to any learned component?

Women may be more likely to report pain than men, including a greater frequency, duration and severity (Unruh 1996), and experimental studies of sex difference in pain have suggested that tolerance of experimentally induced sensory pain may be greater in men (Rollman and Harris 1987; Feine and Bushnell 1991). Social learning has been raised earlier in this chapter as a factor involved with pain, and it becomes relevant in the consideration of any male:female difference. To add to the picture, social learning may bring about a particular way of dealing with pain, while operant conditioning may strengthen this. In the context of pain, and in some stereotyped perspectives, being a man may be associated with stoicism and courage in the face of pain, while women may have been seen as likely to be frail in their response. Each in its own way may meet with reinforcement, whether this comes from family, peers or even health professionals. Whatever the sex of the pain sufferer, stoicism may meet with both positive reinforcement – say, admiration, plus negative reinforcement – avoidance of fuss or undue attention. Frailty and overt suffering may, in a similar way, meet with the positive reinforcement of increased attention, plus the negative reinforcement of avoidance of tasks or responsibilities. Otto and Dougher (1985) examined the relationship between gender and pain response, using masculinity – femininity and social desirability scales. They found that male participants' scores were significantly correlated with pain, with high masculinity scores emerging as associated with elevated pain thresholds.

As with the question of ethnicity, it is the entrenched or stereotyped view which one would hope to avoid. It may be more sensible in practice to envisage the male and female sexes as more alike than they are different, in that each group contains a collection of unique human beings with an individual response to pain.

Physiological sex differences which may impact on pain response have been demonstrated. Sex hormones, naturally, circulate at different levels in men and women, although testosterone is present in women, and oestrogen and progesterone in men. Gear et al. (1996) examined the effect of analgesic drugs on pain related to dental surgery, and found specific drugs to be more effective in women than in men, suggesting a physical difference and including the possibility that testosterone might have a reducing effect, oestrogen a potentiating effect for some analgesics. In premenopausal women a natural and regular fluctuation occurs across the menstrual cycle, allowing research to reveal possible effects of oestrogen and progesterone on pain. Thus studies have been able to show, for example, such findings as greater sensitivity to painful stimuli in women during the luteal phase of their menstrual cycle – that is, in the days after ovulation and prior to menstruation (Tassorelli et al. 2002), and also variation of chronic pain associated with the menstrual cycle (Hellstrom and Anderberg 2003).

Hormonal fluctuations are also thought to influence inflammatory or degenerative processes in certain diseases, thereby impacting on pain report. For example in multiple sclerosis it has been suggested that pregnancy may have a moderating effect on relapsing-remitting form of the disease (Confavreux et al. 1998), while oestrogen and progesterone levels across the menstrual cycle may have an influence on disease activity (Pozzilli et al. 1999). In rheumatoid arthritis too there may be a hormonal effect, and patients may report improvement and associated pain reduction during pregnancy (Forger et al. 2005). The relationship between hormones, stress and rheumatoid arthritis have been discussed previously in Chapter 3.

There is evidence, then, that a variety of factors related to mind and behaviour might affect a person's perception of their pain. This has led to a more holistic approach to pain management, where treatment of underlying disease or condition and administration of analgesic drugs, by whatever route, may be augmented by other approaches. Although it is beyond the scope of this chapter to explore these in detail, there are several interventions, rooted in psychology, which may offer relief to the patient in chronic pain. As outlined earlier in the chapter, the seminal work of Fordyce in 1976 showed how operant or instrumental conditioning – concepts from the behaviourist perspective – might be applied to explain the reinforcement of patterns of pain behaviour. It follows that an operant learning model could be used in an attempt to reshape pain behaviour and increase activity. In a systematic review of the efficacy of behavioural treatments for low back pain, Van Tulder et al. (2000) found an indication that behavioural approaches could have a moderate effect on pain intensity, although less of an effect on functional status – that is, on quality of life factors such as physical, emotional and social aspects.

In contrast, a solely cognitive approach to pain management would mean a different approach. In psychology, the cognitive perspective encompasses a vast range of mental processes, including such things as memory, problem solving, perception and mental representations. For the pain patient, cognitions such as the experience and meaning of pain, or expectations and a sense of control, may be modified by the use of cognitive techniques. Cognitive restructuring (Ellis 1969) might help to ameliorate the pain experience, particularly for the chronic pain sufferer who, realistically, may need to deal with a certain degree of pain for life. By helping the patient with pain to recognise beliefs and thoughts relating to the whole pain experience, cognitive restructuring may result in reframed thinking and a more adapted approach to the situation.

Cognitive behavioural therapy (CBT) – which as the name suggests employs a combination of the two strategies – is an approach which is used now in a number of conditions which involve and impact upon mental health, including anxiety, depression, social phobia and eating disorders. Its main tenet is that an individual's thoughts, beliefs and assumptions and their resultant behaviours can with help or therapy be modified, with a resulting change to their life. CBT may be offered to patients suffering from chronic pain, with a view to helping them to restructure their thoughts and manage their expectations of themselves and their pain. In conjunction with this approach, and depending upon their specialised experience, pain therapy teams may employ additional techniques such as imagery and visualisation.

Such approaches are raised and outlined here simply as a guide to the reader, who may wish to refer to Price and Bushnell (2004) or Schofield (2005) for much more comprehensive discussion.

Conclusion

- Many of the concepts introduced to this chapter will be familiar to practitioners who have undergone programmes of study for health professional registration; psychology is now a common component of the curriculum for the majority of these courses.
- An understanding of pain is invaluable to healthcare practitioners given the importance of pain as a symptom.
- The body of pain psychology literature is immense, and this has been an attempt to draw out a range of points which will be relevant to, and hopefully enhance, the practice of the reader.

References

Aloisi A. and Bonifazi M. (2006) Sex hormones, central nervous system and pain. *Hormones and Behaviour* 50(1): 1–7.
Bandura A., Ross D. and Ross S. (1961) Transmission of aggression through imitation of aggressive models. *Journal of Abnormal and Social Psychology* 63: 575–82.

Barash P., Cullen B. and Stoelting R. (eds) (2006) *Clinical Anaesthesia*, 5th edn. Philadelphia: Lippincott, Williams and Wilkins.

Beecher H. (1956) Relationship of significance of wound to pain experienced. *Journal of the American Medical Association* 161: 1609–13.

Brena S.E. and Chapman S.L. (1985) Acute versus chronic pain states: the Learned Pain Syndrome. *Clinics in Anaesthesiology* 3: 41–55.

Campbell C., Robinson C., Logan M. et al. (2008) Ethnic differences in the nociceptive flexion reflex. *Pain* 134(1–2): 91–6.

Chapman C. (1984) New directions in the understanding and management of pain. *Social Science Medicine* 19(12): 1261–77.

Confavreux C., Hutchinson M., Martine M. et al. (1998) Rate of pregnancy related relapse in multiple sclerosis. *New England Journal of Medicine* 339: 285–91.

Davitz J. and Davitz L. (1981[1901]) *Inferences of patients' pain and psychological distress – studies in nursing behaviour*. New York: Springer.

Ellis A. (1969) A cognitive approach to behaviour therapy. *International Journal of Psychotherapy* 8: 896–900.

Feine J. and Bushnell M. (1991) Sex differences in perception of noxious heat stimuli. *Pain* 44(3): 255–62.

Fordyce W.E. (1976) *Behavioral Methods for Chronic Pain and Illness*. St. Louis, MO: Mosby.

Forger F., Ostensen M., Schumacher A. and Villiger P.M. (2005) Impact of pregnancy on health related quality of life evaluated prospectively in pregnant women with rheumatic diseases by the SF-36 health survey. *Annals of Rheumatic Diseases* 64(10): 1494–9.

Gear R., Miaskowski C., Gordon N. et al. (1996) Kappa-opioids produce significantly greater analgesia in women than in men. *Nature Medicine* 2: 1248–50.

Goldscheider A. (1894) *Ueber den schmerz in Physiologischer und Klinischer Hinsicht*. Berlin: Hirschwald, pp. 1–66.

Greenwald H.P. (1991) Interethnic differences in pain perception. *Pain* 44: 157–63.

Hellstrom B. and Anderberg U. (2003) Pain perception across the menstrual cycle phases in women with chronic pain. *Perceptual and Motor Skills* 96: 201–11.

Hellstrom B. and Erberg U. (2003) Pain perception across the menstrual cycle phases in women with chronic pain. *Perceptual and Motor Skills* 96: 201–11.

Hippocrates, in Peterson W.F. (1946) *Hippocratic wisdom. a modern appreciation of ancient medical science*. Chambers.

Horn S. and Munafo M. (1997) *Pain. Theory, Research and Intervention*. Buckingham: Open University Press.

Hughes J., Smith T. and Kosterlitz H. (1975) Identification of two related pentapeptides from the brain with potent opioid agonist activity. *Nature* 258: 577–9.

Lasch K.E. (2000) Culture, pain, and culturally sensitive pain care. *Pain Management Nursing* 1(Suppl 1): 16–22.

Main C., Sullivan M. and Watson P. (2008) *Pain Management: practical applications of the biopsychosocial perspective in clinical and occupational settings.* Edinburgh: Churchill Livingstone, Elsevier.

Melzack R. and Wall P. (1965) Pain mechanisms: a new theory. *Science* 150: 971–9.

Morrow G. and Dobkin P. (1988) Anticipatory nausea and vomiting in cancer patients undergoing chemotherapy treatment: prevalence, aetiology and behavioural interventions. *Clinical Psychology Review* 85(5): 17–56.

Orwell G. (1949) *Nineteen Eighty-four* Part 3, Chapter 1. London: Martin, Secker and Warburg.

Osgood P.F. and Szyfelbein S. (1989) Management of burn pain in children. *Paediatric Clinics of North America* 36: 1001–12.

Otto M. and Dougher M. (1985) Sex differences and personality factors in responsivity to pain. *Perceptual and Motor Skills* 61(3): 83–90.

Patterson D.R. (2005) Behavioral methods for chronic pain and illness: a reconsideration and appreciation. *Rehabilitation Psychology* 50(3): 312–15.

Pavlov I. (1927) *Conditioned Reflexes.* Translated by G.V. Anrep. Oxford: Oxford University Press.

Pozzilli C., Falaschi P., Mainero C., Martocchia A., D'Urso R., Proietti A., Frontoni M., Bastianello S. and Filippi M. (1999) MRI in multiple sclerosis during the menstrual cycle: relationship with sex hormone patterns. *Neurology* 53(3): 622–4.

Price D. (1988) *Psychological and Neural Mechanisms of Pain.* New York: Raven Press.

Price D. (1999) Psychological mechanisms of pain and analgesia: *Progress in pain research and management Volume 15.* Seattle: IASP Press.

Price D. and Bushnell C. (2004) Psychological methods of pain control: basic science and clinical perspectives: *Progress in pain research and management Volume 29.* Seattle: IASP Press.

Price D., Barrell J. and Gracely R. (1980) A psychophysical analysis of experiential factors that selectively influence the affective dimension of pain. *Pain* 8: 137–49.

Price D.D., Harkins S.W. and Baker C. (1987) Sensory-affective relationships among different types of clinical and experimental pain. *Pain* 28(3): 297–307.

Rollman G. and Harris G. (1987) The detectability, discriminability and perceived magnitude of painful electric shock. *Perception and Psychophysics* 42(3): 257–68.

Rhudy J.L. and Meagher M.W. (2001) The role of emotion in pain modulation. *Current Opinion in Psychiatry* 14: 241–5.

Salmon P. (1990) Women's anticipation and experience of childbirth: the independence of fulfilment, unpleasantness and pain. *British Journal of Medical Psychology* 63: 255–9.

Schneider D. and Palomba H. (2004) Pavlovian conditioning of muscular responses in chronic pain patients: central and peripheral correlates. *Pain* 112(3): 239–47.

Schofield P. (ed.) (2005) *Beyond Pain*. Gateshead: Athenaeum Press.

Skinner B.F. (1953) *Science and Human Behavior*. New York: Free Press.

Snyder S.H., Pert C.B. and Pasternak G.W. (1974) The opiate receptor. *Annals of Internal Medicine* 81(4): 534–40.

Sternbach R.A. and Tursky B. (1965) Ethnic differences among housewives in psychophysical and skin potential responses to electric shock. *Psychophysiology* 1: 241–6.

Tassorelli C., Sandrini G., Cecchini A., Nappi R., Sances G. and Martignoni E. (2002) Changes in nociceptive flexion reflex threshold across the menstrual cycle in healthy women. *Psychosomatic Medicine* 64: 621–6.

Todd K.H., Deaton C., D'Adamo A.P. and Goe L. (2000) Ethnicity and analgesic practice. *Annals of Emergency Medicine* 35(1): 11–6.

Tortora G. and Aganostakis N. (1990) *Principles of Anatomy and Physiology*. New York: Harper Row.

Unruh A.M. (1996) Gender variations in clinical pain experience. *Pain* 65: 123–67.

van Tulder M.W., Ostelo R., Vlaeyen J.W., Linton S.J., Morley S.J. and Assendelft W.J. (2000) B1ehavioral treatment for chronic low back pain: a systematic review within the framework of the Cochrane Back Review Group. *Spine* 25(20): 2688–99.

Von Frey M. (1894) Beitrage zur Physiologie des Schmerzsinnes. *Bericht uber die Verhandlung der koniglichen sachsiger Gesellschaft der Wissenschaften zu Leipzig, mathematisch-physiologische Klasse* 46: 185–96.

Wade J., Dougherty L., Hart R., Rafii A. and Price D. (1992) A canonical correlation analysis of the influence of neuroticism and extraversion on chronic pain, suffering and pain behaviour. *Pain* 5(1): 67–73.

Wall P. (2000) *Pain: the Science of Suffering*. London: Phoenix.

Waters S., Campbell L., Keefe F. and Carson J. (2004) The essence of cognitive-behavioural pain management. In R. Dworkin and W. Breitbart (eds) *Psychosocial Aspects of Pain: a handbook for health care providers*. Seattle: IASP Press.

Weddell G. (1955) Somasthesis and the chemical senses. *Annual Review of Psychology* 6: 119–36.

Zborowski M. (1952) Cultural components of the response to pain. *Journal of Social Issues* 8: 16–30.

Zborowski M. (1969) *People in Pain*. San Francisco: Jossey Bass.

Chapter 5

The pressures and effect of a 'global beauty culture'

Jo Gilmartin

Introduction

The rising tide of body image psychology is steadily increasing, and likely to continue. Other tides rise slowly, whereas the body image construct is powerful and persistent. Overwhelmingly the growth is influenced by changing beauty standards associated with media expectations (Engelin-Maddox 2006), health and diet industries, and cosmetic and bariatric surgery (Herpertz et al. 2003). Most attention is focused on the female body but ideals for men that were formerly 'undeveloped' are now going through a major shift. Researchers appear to conceptualise the body image dynamic on a process continuum, with levels of dissatisfaction ranging from benign to extreme. Typically, lower levels of disturbance are linked to self-esteem concerns, higher levels associated with anxiety, depression and a poor sense of well-being. Discourses on moderate levels of body image dissatisfaction make their appeal strongly, held in an 'ikon' of enlightenment leading to healthy exercise and eating patterns (Bordo 2003; Weaver and Byers 2006). In the lower to moderate categories there appears to be a sense of transcendence and new possibility, as if the chains can be removed. This chapter, then, is concerned with body image, media representations and effect. The problem of eating disorders will be considered too, pointing to interventions for promoting positive health.

Media representation and body image ideals

Disturbance in body image attitude comes from dissatisfaction with appearance and, paradoxically, makes anxieties about body image a central defining feature of self or self-identity. Body dissatisfaction represents a major psychological discrepancy between perceived body and ideal body (Halliwell and Dittmar 2006). This can have significant effects in influencing negative self-beliefs and unhealthy body shaping behaviours. Thus a higher investment in appearance, especially when the actual body size is discrepant to the sociocultural body ideal, is usually linked to lower satisfaction (Cash et al. 2004). Dissatisfaction with and overvaluation of appearance are key factors in the development of eating disorders (Dokter 2000) and body dysmorphic disorder (Veale 2004). Therefore, it is essential to penetrate the veil of dissatisfaction in attempting to understand body image psychology.

Media representation of increasingly thinner body shape gains supremacy in the discourse of women. Heightened body dissatisfaction appears to be a growing trend amongst adolescent girls. This preoccupation frequently disguises the fact that men, too, are defined by their bodies. James (2007) poses an important question – are you infected with affluenza? He suggests that the 'affluenza virus' is a set of values concerned with acquiring material possessions, body image and fame which increases susceptibility to emotional distress, depression, anxiety, substance abuse and personality disorder. The epidemic of 'affluenza' is spreading globally and deserves closer inspection in the context of media influence.

Women and women's bodies

One crucial factor negatively affecting the body image satisfaction of women is the media ideal of thinness, which glorifies it as a vital ingredient of beauty and success, denigrating fatness by linking it to negative characteristics such as ugliness, laziness and failure (Rothblum 1994). Several studies have demonstrated that exposure to thin media images markedly lowers body image satisfaction (Bessenoff 2006; Engelin-Maddox 2006; Ginsberg and Gray 2006). Typically, athletes who read judged sports magazines (*USA Gymnastics*) are exposed to thinner cover models than those reading non-judged ones (*Golf for Women*) (Ginsberg and Gray 2006). The social comparison process encourages athletes to aspire to and physically look like the cover models, leading to body image dissatisfaction and restricted eating behaviour. Many studies now exist demonstrating the relationship between exercise and eating disorders in the elite athlete (Hulley and Hill 2001). Distance runners, for example, demand a thin body build and show a higher than expected prevalence of eating disorders. Women's magazines focus explicitly on 'glamour', 'body shape', 'looking sexy', 'diet products' and 'cosmetic surgery', offering humorous but contradictory messages. These glossies offer many flawed narratives to teenagers and women seeking self-improvement and well-being leading to inner turmoil and unrealistic fantasies.

The growing discrepancy in appearance between average women and media ideals may account for body image disturbance, eating dysfunction and lowered self-esteem. Increased cultural expectations of thinness are evidenced by the decreasing size of women displayed in the popular media (Wykes and Gunter 2006). Women are encouraged to engage in unhealthy eating and exercise habits in an effort to achieve this ideal (see Table 5.1). This is equally well forecast in Engelin-Maddox (2006). Media ideals become imperative, as women

Table 5.1 The consequences of media print for women

Type	Message	Consequence
Magazines	Thinness associated with success and beauty	Normative weight dissatisfaction and body image disturbance
	Fatness linked with characteristics of ugliness, laziness and failure	Stigmatisation and maltreatment of obese people
		Fantasies about cosmetic surgery and possible eating disorders
	Thinness, fitness and high energy associated with power, resilience and creativity	Increases the significance of vital energy and well-being
	Unhealthy messages about eating and dieting	Regimes of dieting and exercise with the potential to trigger eating disorders
	'Chic', fashionable, glamorous, gorgeous and glad to be gay	Stereotypes images of women in general
Soaps	Rigid and narrow messages about attractiveness	Increased negative moods, levels of depression and lowered self-esteem
Visual media	Stereotypes of thinness and body ideal	Influences beliefs in optimal body image/appearance
	Thinner models associated with fame	Drive to thinness and body image dissatisfaction
Cinema	Fanged Vampire (The Hunger) Chic femme beauty (Les Bides) Depressed loner (Rachel, Rachel)	Stereotypes gay women
	Mrs Henderson/The new James Bond (gorgeous Judy Dench)	Optimism, hope and the ultimate source of mid-life beauty

show no interest in challenging the appearance of stereotypes associated with beauty. Arguably, however, not all women are significantly affected by such messages. Reactions to the thin ideal may be moderated by variables such as external pressures to be thin, body dissatisfaction and social support (Weaver and Byers 2006). To counter this superficial approach, feminist writers have attempted to return to the structural, cultural and economic ways in which our bodies are produced (Grosz and Probyn 1996; Lumby and Probyn 2003).

Fashion photography frequently displays the lookalike bodies of female models to sell clothes with subtle suggestions of anorexic desire. By contrast, lesbians are depicted by the popular press in a number of bizarre stereotypes such as 'heavily muscled and single breasted' or 'bra burning amazons' (Creed 1996: 86). In paintings, women often appear with 'identical faces, hair, clothes', locked in a close embrace (Creed 1996). Nevertheless, there is evidence to suggest that lesbians are less influenced by sociocultural norms of thinness and have a more positive view of overweight female bodies. Unlike heterosexual women, they appear to possess a more flexible outlook of the female body (Morrison et al. 2004), which renders them less susceptible to negative body image and less likely to aspire to the ideal.

Men's bodies

Body image studies among men demonstrate the same media image ideals as for women in terms of physique and attractiveness. Men's bodies are treated equally as objects to be gazed upon. Crucially, the media impact should take into account the masculine self-perception benchmark. The gay male culture appears to endorse the stereotype that gay men are more appearance orientated than heterosexual men (Tiggemann et al. 2007). A survey undertaken by Levesque and Vichesky (2006) assessed the nature and correlates of body image dissatisfaction among 64 gay men. The survey focused on assessments such as perceived acceptance within the gay community, social comparison tendencies, body image satisfaction, self-esteem and depression. The results indicated that the participants had relatively positive self-esteems but the social comparison related to less body satisfaction. Most valued and desired muscular physiques ($M = 4.29$, $SD = 1.34$). In contrast to women, gay men seem to be primarily interested in gaining weight by developing muscularity. Heavier gay men appear also to want to reduce body fat and gain muscle. Overall, the pursuit of muscularity seemed more significant for gay men than heterosexual men (Table 5.2).

Table 5.2 The consequences of media print for men

Type	Message	Consequence
Magazines	Muscular and V-shaped-sexy, healthy and powerful	Normative discontent for gay men in particular
		Drive to reduce body fat and increase well-being
		Drive to body building
	Fatness linked to potential health problems and lack of sexual prowess	Emotional distress and anxiety
		Stigmatisation and social exclusion
	Gay grooming and youthful beauty	Stereotypes gay men
	Hair loss, bulges and bumps as characteristics of unattractiveness	Increased body image dissatisfaction, lowered self-esteem
	Body building, dieting, plastic surgery and calf implants, to achieve ideal physique	Fantasies about cosmetic surgery
Visual media	Muscular physique, strong	Obsessive dieting, exercising and body building
	Efficacious and physically fit	Stereotypes strong muscular physique with aggressive traits
	Adiposity associated with lack of will/sloppiness	Body image disturbance
Cinema	Tall, fit and handsome men represent fame/power	Internalisation of media ideas as significant
	Eschew small, energised men with notably less beauty and power	Biased social and sexual fantasies concerning beauty and power

Superficially, these aspirations of muscularity seem to indicate the pleasures offered by the masculine space. However, the use of the body against the threat of ageing is not clearly defined amongst gay men. The images depicted in the gay media largely represent young bodies; hence being youthful may be integral to the gay ideal as much as being muscular and slim (Mann 1988). In effect, gay men have similar expectations as women in terms of muscularity, youth and beauty. Moreover, the media and the Internet highlight programmes that emphasise dieting and male muscularity, featuring body building, dieting, plastic surgery and calf implants, to achieve an ideal physique. This can trigger illusions about normal bodies. Contemporary associations of obesity depicted in the media are not focused on the accumulation of wealth for men, but perhaps reflect moral or personal inadequacy or lack of will. Adiposity is a major challenge for men because media images of male bodies have become increasingly 'muscular and V-shaped, emphasising broad shoulders, developed arms and chest muscles, and slim waists' (Schooler and Ward 2006: 2). This meso-morphic (muscular build) body type has surged in media portrayals triggering increasing body image dissatisfaction amongst gay and heterosexual men (Tiggemann et al. 2007). Muscularity is tied to cultural meanings, which view men to be powerful, strong, efficacious and physically fit. But at the same time, muscularity has been associated with amateur status, the insensitive, unintelligent, physically abusive and uncultured body typology (Bordo 2003).

The Internet

The web is another powerful medium, particularly important for our analysis. The form is not substantially different in content from previous media forms. Wykes and Gunter (2006: 121) suggest that in many respects it is 'more ready, accessible and multi-layered in representation – sound, graphic, video, image and text are possible in one message, integrating advertising with entertainment and information'. Electronic magazines construct the female body and the male muscular physique in the same vein as depicted in hard copies on the shop shelves (*Marie Clare, Glamour, Vogue, Men's Fitness, Diva, Bent, Attitudes*). Typically, websites generate bodies of knowledge despite lack of control or ownership, reflecting dominant interests, and often subtly justifying the status quo. This unregulated information can be extremely dangerous in regard to pro-anorexia websites with 'thinspiration' targeted at teenagers. Crucially, healthcare providers need to be aware of the 'tips and tricks' of such websites that endorse the practice of anorexia behaviour (Norris et al. 2006).

Certainly, the contemporary standard of beauty in relation to body shape is broadcast by the major mass media. The social comparison process helps to explain how human beings have an innate tendency to make comparisons in an effort to self-evaluate. This is often further compounded by internalisation of 'ideal' images that place pressure on both women and men to conform to body image representations that are currently in vogue.

It is not, however, only media representation that jars badly. Surprisingly, only a small number of individuals question the authority of the media and the inhumane aspects of its interjects. It is perhaps at the intersection between the media ideal and the construction of appearance schema that the assumed contribution of men and women is raised. More fascinating is the discursive production of different cultural/gendered expectations and the subjectivities that get constructed as a result.

Despite dominant media ideals and gendered body image, such ideals are arguably extremely narrow and rigid; historical configurations become obsolete. In many respects, this old-fashioned culture is drenched in alienation, persecution and misery. Therefore, it is important to break the associations between gendered body image and appearance ideals and to radically rethink what we want the fit, agile, healthy, idiosyncratic body image to be.

Modern print: selling slenderness to teenagers

Body image dissatisfaction may be established in both female and male teenagers aged 13 years, posing a risk factor for the development of eating disorders (Gehrman et al. 2006). This section will trace the cause and growth of some disturbances. Modern print media including the teen magazines *Como-girl*, *Sugar*, *Bliss*, *J17* and *Shape* focus on beauty, fashion, sex, dieting, cool celebrities, shopping, and slenderness and attracting the opposite sex. There is some evidence to suggest that teenage magazines construct a seductive meaning of an aesthetic gaze that is sexually desirable (Wykes and Gunter 2006). Teenage girls often grow up with enlightenment or fear regarding body image. They seek out possibilities and reassurances from glossy magazines about the new or ideal self. The deconstruction of different meanings has the capacity to stir up diverse fantasies and images for the contemporary culture. The process is frequently marked with the tyranny of slimness and body objectification leading to body dissatisfaction and low self-esteem (Table 5.3). Social stereotyping of body shapes is prominent among teenagers. Obese and overweight body shapes tend to be portrayed in negative terms whereas slender body shapes are construed as attractive among members of the same and opposite sex (Collins 1991).

One significant factor of potential media influence is the extent to which girls make comparisons to celebrities featured in sleek magazines. Bessenoff (2006) undertook an exploration of body image self-discrepancy and social comparison in the effects on women from thin-ideal media images. This experimental study included 112 female psychology undergraduates. The women with high and low body image self-discrepancy were exposed to advertisements either with thin women (thin-ideal) or without thin women (neutral-advertisement control). The results showed that exposure to thin-ideal advertisements increased body image dissatisfaction, negative mood, levels of depression and lowered self-esteem. Body image self-discrepancy generally

Table 5.3 Teenage slenderness – causation and impact on body image

Causation	Message	Impact
Glossy magazines	Slimness is the beauty ideal	Emotional distress and poor self-esteem
	Distorted information on dieting, health and fitness	Preoccupied with limiting their diet
	Slim figures attract the opposite sex	Body image dissatisfaction
	Highlight plastic surgery to achieve a beautiful body	Disturbance in developing self-identity
TV adverts	Promote slim women as sex objects – body objectification	Increased body dissatisfaction Low self-esteem
Music videos	Promote thin, attractive models	Increased body dissatisfaction among teenagers
Photographs of models	Normalise an illusion of desirable bodies	Increased eating disorders Social comparisons Disturbance in psychosexual development
Sports-gymnasts, rowers, runners	Leanness dependent sports encourage weight reduction	Restricted eating Increased anorexia tendencies
Cultural and social factors	Attitudes influence the beauty benchmark	Agitated behaviour, mood swings
	Intrusive parenting, poses difficulty for developing adolescents to become autonomous	Pursuit of thinness, exertion of personal control

moderated these effects. Typically, women with high self-discrepancy levels experienced higher levels of dejection, agitation-related mood and lowered self-esteem when they viewed the thin-ideal advertisements. Contrastingly, the women with low body-image levels did not show these differences.

Groesz et al. (2002) have completed a particularly useful meta-analysis of 25 experimental studies that examine exposure to media images on body satisfaction. The results showed that body image was significantly more negative after viewing thin media images in comparison to viewing average size models, plus size models or inanimate objects. This negative impact was more marked amongst adolescent girls under 19 years old, and for those who are vulnerable to thin media models. This finding clearly supports the sociocultural viewpoint that the mass media transmit a slender ideal that draws out body dissatisfaction.

Teenagers who agonise about ideal body shape often become preoccupied with dieting. Eating behaviour is sometimes triggered by diet information found in glossy magazines and many teenagers wish to imitate models. This is further compounded by the fact that girls enter a patriarchal world in which they are expected to behave in 'feminine' ways in their relationships and confirm to media images of beauty. This dilemma has been most clearly explained by the feminist psycho-dynamic perspective. Orbach (1978) outlines the characteristics of successful femininity including anticipating and meeting the needs of others, deferring to others and seeking self-definition through others. The major consequence is that women often deny themselves, and teenagers in particular are often unable to develop an authentic sense of need, feeling and desire.

Moreover, this socially constructed, oppressive ideology (Friere 1970) influences female adolescent development with possible implications for mental health and well-being. There is also evidence to suggest that body objectification is related to factors such as body esteem, body shame (Noll and Frederickson 1998) and disordered eating (Slater and Tiggemann 2002). Bordo (2003) points to the visual theme in teenagers' magazines of women hiding in the shadows of men, seeking solace in their arms. These images uphold traditional gender relations and perhaps sustain oppression.

There is a growing body of research evidence that music videos have a significant impact on adolescents. Bell et al. (2007) designed an exposure experiment that examined the impact of thin models in music videos on body dissatisfaction of 87 adolescent girls aged 16–19 years. Under the guise of a memory experiment, 30 girls were exposed to music videos highlighting thin, attractive models, 30 listened to music video songs, and 27 were asked to learn a list of 20 neutral words. Of the three interventions, the girls who watched the music videos reported significantly elevated scores on an adaptation of the Body Image States Scale, signifying increased body dissatisfaction. Furthermore, this negative impact of music television on body dissatisfaction was also emphasised by Tiggemann and Slater (2004).

Consistent research evidence documents that appearance related concerns are troublesome for teenagers. The Tolman et al. (2006) study examined femininity ideology and adolescent girls' mental health using a survey instrument. One hundred and forty-eight girls aged 12 to 15 years completed the survey. The sample was diverse in terms of ethnicity and race including 52% white, 20% Latino, 16% multiracial, 4% black, 3% Asian and 5% other/missing. The results showed that body objectification and, to a lesser extent, authenticity in relationships explained half the variance of depression and over two-thirds of self-esteem in a critical period of development for adolescents. This study focuses specifically on girls and femininity but excludes masculine ideologies, which might be useful.

Fitness activities

For boys, there are circumstances where sports participation is a risk factor particularly in the development of eating disorders. A crucial fact is that anorexia athletica is common in leanness-dependent and weight-dependent sports (Sundgot-Borgen and Torstveit 2004). Reducing weight can provide a competitive edge in gymnasts, wrestlers, runners, body builders, rowers, jockeys, dancers and ski-jumpers. They are often influenced by intense pressure from competitive coaches, team-mates, and parents. Hatmaker (2006) suggests that boys who are involved in sports that require large or muscular physiques often use performance-enhancing drugs such as steroids, human growth hormone and nutritional supplements. Interestingly, gay boys are at greater risk of developing eating disorders in comparison with heterosexual men. Moreover, Fichter and Daser (1987) reported that homosexuality, bisexuality and transgender seem to pose a risk factor for eating disorders.

Difficult and unexpected feelings are sometimes aroused for girls in relation to sporting activities. The media transmit powerful messages designed to promote exercise and fitness. Thus, the weight control benefits of fitness are usually associated with beauty. However, there are stigmas connected with sports and fitness activities that collide with the portrayal of a beautiful body image. Indeed, sporting activities can increase body temperature, sweat release and unpleasant odours, which can conflict with looking gorgeous. Additionally, participating in sports might involve undressing or wearing clothes that reveal body shape to peers and significant others. This is potentially humiliating for teenagers who are self-conscious.

Cultural and social factors

The mass media also influence cultural and social factors in relation to perceptions of body image. A cross-sectional study of 447 Bahraini male and female adolescents aged 12–17 was undertaken by Al-Sendi et al. (2004), focusing on body weight perception. Attitude measures, including those of parents and friends, were employed towards their weight status. Silhouette illustrations were used to measure perception of ideal body image. The results showed that teenagers tended to underestimate their weight status, particularly among the overweight and obese. Approximately half the girls and one third of the boys disclosed discontent with their current body weight. Interestingly, the Bahraini adolescents' weight-related beliefs and attitudes appear to fall at two ends of the spectrum: a tolerance of obesity at one end and contrastingly an exaggerated concern for its occurrence at the other.

The study of culture and religion is taken a step further amongst Arab schoolgirls in Israel. Latzer et al. (2007) examined the prevalence of eating disorder behaviour among three specific religious sub-groups. The sample involved 1,131 adolescents, including 922 (81.5%) Moslem, 125 (11.1%) Christian, and 84 (7.4%) Druze. The results displayed a significantly lower eating disorder total amongst the Christian subgroup. Remarkably, the Moslem and Druze had similar eating disorder inventory-2 (ED1–2) scores. One possible explanation for this result is that the Moslem population in Israel often has problems with self-esteem (Azaiza and Ben Ari 1998). Contrastingly, Christians appear to be better educated and enjoy a higher socio-economic status.

Eating disorders are often construed as obsessional behaviour, associated with dependence in opposition to independence and mothering issues (Winnicott 1965). Representations in the media strongly influence social and cultural factors, hence parenting styles. Intrusive or over-protective parental interjects can pose difficulty for the developing adolescent to become autonomous. Thus, the pursuit of thinness is an exertion of personal control leading to increased anorexic tendencies. Power and voice are mediated with the body. Interestingly, Lee and Lock (2007) reported that Asian-American adolescents scored lower on the eating disorder examination (EDE) subscale, significantly on the restraint subscale (1.48 vs. 2.80, p = 0.016) and weight concerns subscale (1.35 vs. 2.30, p = 0.026) in comparison with a non-Asian sample. The validity of this finding is questionable. Lee and Lock (2007: 230) go on to suggest that 'denial of symptoms is common in anorexia nervosa among Asians because many are culturally encouraged to use minimization to cope with taboo conditions'.

For teenagers at a global level the body is a powerful symbolic form, operating as a symbol for culture and a direct locus of social control. This contemporary aesthetic ideal has become an obsessive pursuit tormenting many teenagers' lives, thus leaving many teenagers vulnerable to external regulation, improvement and transformation. Teenagers need to be encouraged to selectively control their exposure to mediated depictions of an attractiveness ideal and not adhere to media images. Despite cultural norms teenagers need to be encouraged to be self-determining agents, critically appraising media ideals and celebrating their emerging sexuality. It is crucial that they believe in their own personal choices to be an individual, freely motivated and empowered.

Transcending media ideals

One vital ingredient in designing a theoretically sound prevention programme for eating disorders is targeting media portrayals of idealised attractiveness. At the level of research, there is a fairly strong case for the utilisation of a school based media literacy programme and a self-esteem programme for teenagers. Wade et al. (2003) utilised a five-lesson media literacy programme to achieve short-term decreases in weight concern with 13-year-old boys and girls. The interactive, student-centred, self-esteem building framework may perhaps be a safe and effective way of reducing risk factors for eating disorders.

The efficacy of single media literacy lessons in reducing media internalisation in adolescents yielded interesting results (Wilksch et al. 2006). Post-intervention, the girls experienced less impressive statistical improvements than the boys. Perhaps the content and duration of the programme requires careful consideration for optimal benefit for girls and boys. The impact of media literacy programmes as a prevention intervention for eating disorders among college women was examined by Coughlin and Kalodner (2006). The results provide favourable support for such literacy amongst high-risk female college students but long-term follow-up studies are required for a more rigorous evaluation of its efficacy.

This, however, is only a partial answer. The central point is that many forms of intervention might be justifiable. A further strategy is to focus on promoting a healthy lifestyle including nutritional advice and the benefits of exercise. Personal, social and health education (PSHE) and physical education are significant features in the National Curriculum (http://www.nc.uk.net). Although many inspirational teachers attempt to empower children and adolescents to lead healthy and independent lives, parents often negate this knowledge and understanding. This can leave children vulnerable to confusion, emotional distresses and substance abuse.

The slender body and eating disorders

The growing social pressure for a slim body shape has resulted in restrained eating or disturbances that have dramatically increased the prevalence of anorexia, bulimia and other forms of disordered eating. This has become a significant contemporary public health concern. Bordo (2003: 49) suggests that attempts persist to link eating disorders with one specific pathological situation – biological, psychological or familial. Other factors that might contribute to women developing eating disorders include power inequalities, sexism, and the threat of emotional or physical violence and sexual abuse (Lyubomirsky et al. 2001).

Different forms of psychopathology appear to trigger eating disorders and include irritable moods, depression, neuroticism and insecure attachments (Eggert et al. 2007). Feminists in particular are sensitive about the associations of eating disorders with middle-class families. Probyn (2007) claims that anorexia is constructed as glamorous in the new media (www.wun.ac.uk gender network). This particular representation has its problems. For instance, if glamorous values are allowed to pass into the public sphere as legitimate forms of being, this force will increasingly further erode self-conception and body image issues. Accumulating evidence suggests that the contributors and triggers of eating disorders are multidimensional 'becoming less and less amenable to scientific clarity and distinctiveness' (Bordo 2003: 49).

Anorexia nervosa

Orbach (2006: 151) noted that people who suffer from anorexia nervosa 'express their preoccupation with food by becoming very thin and sometimes to the point of death through starvation'. Some people with anorexia nervosa engage in eating binges. This process is often followed by self-disgust that drives the sufferer to take laxatives, to fast and to vomit. Two distinct subtypes of anorexia nervosa have been identified (Roth and Fonagy 2006: 236): either regular binge eating or purging, or the restrictive type, where these behaviours are not present. Anorexia nervosa generally begins in adolescence with a high prevalence of body discontent experienced by girls. Roth and Fonagy (2006) note that bimodal peaks occur at the ages of 14 and 18 years. Some data predict a good recovery rate, others point to continuing disordered eating moving to bulimia patterns or perhaps EDNOS (eating disorders not otherwise specified) (Lowe et al. 2001).

Psychodynamic explanations of anorexia nervosa have alluded to troublesome early mother–child relations that have impaired the child's capacity to establish a distinctive identity. Thus, embellished efforts to control weight symbolise the adolescent struggle to establish a type of unique identity (Palazzoli 1978). Other psychoanalysts perceive anorexia nervosa as representing a typical regression to a more primitive stage of development amongst people who cannot cope with the challenges of growing up (Szyrynski 1973). The adolescent is often torn by conflicting and contradictory demands particularly at the onset of puberty and with the physical and psychological changes that it holds.

Bulimia

As a disorder, bulimia, or the dietary chaos syndrome (Berkman et al. 2007), is behaviourally manifest in the consumption of large quantities of food, perhaps in eating 'binges', with lack of control over eating behaviour. This is usually followed by self-induced efforts to purge the food by vomiting, the utilisation of laxatives or diuretics, fasting or over-exercising. Typically, these episodes might occur at least three times per week. Hallings-Pott et al. (2005) report dissociative states surrounding binge episodes, for example, depersonalisation or feeling dazed. The western culture drive to the thinness and beauty ideal might overwhelm women and consequently some desire to 'escape' or disso-ciate from the self through binging (Everill et al. 1995). Despite the prevalence of health education, bulimia nervosa usually starts in late adolescence or sometimes in early adulthood. This chronic condition is often manifested by episodes of remission and relapse.

Lyubomirsky et al. (2001) examined dissociative experiences and abnormal eating in 92 non-eating-disordered and 61 aged-matched women with bulimia. In the non-clinical sample, dissociative tenden-cies in women who had never been diagnosed with an eating disorder were connected to abnormal eating attitudes and behaviour even after controlling aspects of psychopathology. Pathological variables that were emphasised included sexual abuse, emotional distress and suicide impulses. The results also showed that in both groups a com-bination of both negative-effect and dissociative experiences preceding a binge was linked to the highest levels of abnormal eating. Interest-ingly, in both bulimic and occasional binge eaters, the feeling of panic appeared to decrease as a binge episode progressed, whereas, in bulimic women only, dissociative experiences appeared to increase during binge eating.

Most attention in the evidence-based literature focuses on anorexia and bulimia. However, Roth and Fonagy (2006) go on to suggest that a high percentage of patients present criteria not otherwise specified (EDNOS). In most cases the symptoms resonate on the anorexia or bulimia spectrum, but they do not meet the diagnostic criteria. Despite the 'sub-threshold' from a diagnostic standpoint, their holistic needs might be equivalent to clients meeting the complete criteria for both anorexia and bulimia (Roth and Fonagy 2006: 237).

Shame and eating disorders

Research evidence is beginning to point to the notion of shame, in regard to eating disorders and its disclosure in treatment. Swan and Andrews (2003) explored shame in 68 women who had undergone treatment for eating disorders (EDs) in comparison to 72 non-clinical controls. The mean age of the ED group was 30.76 years and 98% were of white British/European origin. The mean age of the control group was 26.2 years. The participants completed a questionnaire on ED, depressive symptoms, bodily, behavioural and character shame and shame around eating. The results showed that the ED group scored significantly higher than the control one on all shame areas. In addition, a substantial proportion (42%) of the eating disordered participants reported that they had not disclosed the important issue of shame during contact with health professionals. This finding has implications for professionals working clinically with patients with ED, particularly in allowing the exploration of shame in a safe and accepting environment.

Sexual orientation and eating disorders

Prevalence of eating disorders is clearly linked to gay and bisexual populations. Feldman and Myers (2007) undertook a study involving 126 white heterosexuals and 388 white, black, Latino lesbian, gay and bisexual men and women with a diagnosis of anorexia, bulimia and binge eating disorders. The results revealed that gay and bisexual men had a significantly higher prevalence of eating disorders than heterosexual men. There were no differences reported amongst the women.

A particularly interesting piece of research has been recently completed by Wichstrøm (2006) on sexual orientation as a risk factor for bulimic symptoms. This study focused on whether sexual orientation predicts future bulimic symptoms and alternatively alleged that risk factors associated with non-heterosexual sexual orientation explained the increased risk. The sample included Norwegian high school students aged 10 to 14 years (n = 2,924) who completed self-reports about bulimic symptoms including same-sex sexual experiences, degree of sexual attraction to the same sex, and alleged risk factors. The participants were re-examined five years later (T2). The results showed that same-sex sexual experience before T1 increased the prevalence of bulimic symptoms at T2. Males reporting homosexual tendencies at

T1 had higher odds for bulimic symptoms in comparison with hetero-sexual males. This finding concurs with other studies pointing to a higher risk of pathological eating symptoms among non-heterosexual males (Levesque and Vichesky 2006).

Exercise and eating disorders

The relationship between exercise and eating disorder features has been examined by Lipsey et al. (2006). The community sample consisted of adult women with and without eating disorder psychopathology. This study focused on the cognitions of exercisers who scored high and low on eating disorder symptoms. This cross-sectional comparative study recruited a sample of 260 female sports centre users; the mean age was 29.4 years (range 18–63 years). The results showed that the eating disorder psychopathology was associated with commitment to exercise, body weight and depression, suggesting that exercise commitment was linked to weight and mood regulation in women with eating disorder features. These characteristics were not associated with how frequently the women exercised, or the period of their exercise bouts, refuting the idea that psychopathology can be inferred from exercise behaviour alone. Among research published prior to Lipsey et al's. (2006) work, findings point to a similar direction, linking eating disorder psychopathology with commitment to exercise but not to frequency or duration (Adkins and Keel 2005).

Body image disturbance

Eating disorders involve a body image disturbance. The research evidence examined indicates that the degree and form of disturbance can vary among women and men. It can thus take on multidimensional characteristics involving attitudinal, perceptual, emotional and behavioural features. Bordo (2003) noted that the metaphysic of the person with anorexia is associated with Augustine's configuration of the spiritual struggle of the two wills within, a contest between good and evil. Thinness represents a triumph of the will over the body connecting with 'absolute purity and transcendence of the flesh' (Bordo 2003: 148). This dualistic dimension often poses a huge challenge in the contemporary culture with individuals obsessed with the control of the unruly body.

Treatments for eating disorders

Psychological interventions appear to focus on mental health need, which might come either from the effects of, or cause of, the eating disorder. Typically, this includes anxiety, depression, personality disorder, addictive-compulsive behaviour or self-esteem issues. There is an increasing range of individual psychotherapies utilised in the treatment of anorexia nervosa (Roth and Fonagy 2006). This includes behavioural, cognitive behavioural and psychodynamic techniques. Family therapies are popular too, and crucially, establishing dietary advice is a vital ingredient in the treatment process. Treatment is usually aligned to meet individual needs directly related to eating disorder symptoms including dietary advice, medication such as antidepressants and nutritional supplements and a specific psychological intervention.

Given the high morbidity accompanying anorexia nervosa and bulimia, developing effective treatment is vital. Systematic reviews shed light on the efficacy of different forms of psychotherapeutic interventions and family therapy. Despite the huge number of studies undertaken, the research evidence is somewhat ambiguous. In their review, Bulik et al. (2007) reported the beneficial effects from several types of intervention: for example, cognitive behavioural therapy (CBT) significantly reduced relapse risk. Focal family therapy was superior to routine treatment but equivalent to cognitive analytic therapy (CAT) in increasing percentage of adult body weight, and family therapy was more effective for adolescent patients in comparison to older patients with chronic symptoms. Roth and Fonagy (2006) point to the positive effects of cognitive and cognitive behavioural interventions in the improvement of binging and purging (Table 5.4) in people with bulimia, although secondary outcomes such as reduction in body dissatisfaction or lessening in depression and anxiety are not emphasised.

Cognitive behavioural therapy appears to be fairly well established as a useful intervention but it is difficult to evaluate its effectiveness as a valid treatment option for every individual. Given the scope of the cause of eating disorders particularly in relation to psychodynamic variables it is not realistic to expect that CBT is appropriate in every situation. Therefore, it is crucial that health professionals critically appraise the evidence especially in relation to longitudinal studies.

Contrastingly, people with eating disorders frequently experience internal conflict, and some perceive talk therapy as an intrusion. Recognition is slowly dawning that people are enabled to face and work through the anxieties that are mobilised in other forms, for example, the application of art therapy (Schaverin and Rust 2000), dance movement therapy (Totenbier and Payne 2000) or group therapy. In

Table 5.4 Interventions for eating disorders

Intervention	Beneficial effect
Cognitive behavioural therapy (CBT)	Improvement of binging and purging in bulimia Identified dysfunctional beliefs about eating in anorexia Enhanced motivation to change in anorexia patients Patients taught to challenge distorted thoughts
Family therapy	Effective for adolescent patients Established an appropriate dietary regime Resolution of psychological tensions
Cognitive analytic therapy	Improvement of binging and purging in bulimia Weight gain in anorexia patient sustained over 1 year follow up Improvement in eating behaviour
Art therapy	Creative expression of inner conflict Frozen fears about repressed aspects of self might be released Freedom and self understanding might develop
Dance movement therapy	Dancing out through the body underlying emotional conflict Creative engagement with emotions associated with the movement
Relaxation techniques – massage	Psychological effects include release of tension and anxiety, feelings of security and safety, nurturing and feelings of blissfulness

Source: Dokter (2000); Roth and Fonagy (2006)

terms of treatment, evidence shows that both art therapy and dance movement therapy have been useful in NHS psychiatric units (Dokter 2000). People with anorexia, bulimia and compulsive overeating often have huge challenges around the issue of control. They are frequently invaded by distorted feelings about 'self' and 'sense of identity'. Therefore relaxation interventions in the form of massage are indeed powerful in promoting feelings of blissfulness and well-being.

Conclusion

- Challenges have arisen from the media, some emotionally charged, targeted at teenagers searching for identity, 'slimy desires' of the flesh for the obese and muscular perfection for men.
- It is evident from the media that the messages transmitted represent bias towards a very slender female body type or mesomorphic typology for men.

- The body is often experienced as 'alien', 'ugly', exerting a downward pull for people with appearance related concerns. Women in particular appear to aspire to a high self-esteem, which is constantly eroded by obesity and body image issues.
- The ideas portrayed in the media in relation to feminine attractiveness and beauty are narrow and rigid, with a significant emphasis placed on thinness.
- There is a danger that internalisation of media interjects could increase the possibility of eating disorders, especially amongst teenagers.
- Gay men in particular are subjected to body image disturbance following exposure to media print and social expectations.
- Drawing on media print the body ideal portrayed leads to body dissatisfaction, which activates social and inappropriate comparisons, low self-esteem, unhealthy dieting regimes and poor well-being.
- Research evidence points to the effectiveness of educational interventions to help teenagers transcend media ideals, devoting time to discernment, positive coping and creating healthier lifestyles.
- There is a dearth of research to shed light on the impact of educational programmes or new age workshops for adults experiencing body image dissatisfaction.
- Research on interventions to help with eating disorders has focused predominately on the effectiveness of CBT and family therapy. Both appear to be beneficial in the short term.
- More longitudinal research is needed to examine individual variation and progress across the process of a life span.
- Above all else, the pathological implications of appearance ideals portrayed in the media invite us to challenge its authoritarian, disempowering nature, and to construct a fresh understanding of what a healthy, cherished sense of body image might be.

References

Adkins E.C. and Keel P.K. (2005) Does 'excessive' or 'compulsive' best describe exercise as a symptom of bulimia nervosa? *International Journal of Eating Disorders* 38: 24–9.

Al-Sendi A.M., Shetty P. and Musaiger A.O. (2004) Body weight perception among Bahraini adolescents. *Child: Care, Health and Development* 30(4): 369–76.

Azaiza F. and Ben Ari A. (1998) Self perception of minority group adolescents: The experience of Arabs living in Israel. *Scandinavian Journal of Social Welfare* 7: 236–43.

Bell B.T., Lawton R. and Dittmar H. (2007) The impact of thin models in music videos on adolescent girls' body dissatisfaction. *Body Image* 4: 137–45.

Berkman N.D., Lohr K.N. and Bulik C.M. (2007) Outcome of eating disorders: a systematic review of the literature. *International Journal of Eating Disorders* 40(4): 293–309.

Bessenoff G.R. (2006) Can the media affect us? Social comparison, self-discrepancy, and the thin ideal. *Psychology of Women Quarterly* 30: 239–51.

Bordo S. (2003) *Unbearable Weight. Feminism, Western Culture, and the Body*. London: University of California Press.

Bulik C.M., Berkman N.D., Brownley K.A., Sedway J.A. and Lohr K.N. (2007) Anorexia nervosa treatment: a systematic review of randomized controlled trials. *International Journal of Eating Disorders* 40(4): 310–20.

Cash T.F., Melnyk S.E. and Hrabosky J.I. (2004) The assessment of body image investment: an extensive revision of the Appearance Schemas Inventory. *International Journal of Eating Disorders* 35: 305–16.

Collins M. (1991) Body figure perceptions and preferences among preadolescent children. *International Journal of Eating Disorders* 10: 199–208.

Coughlin J.W. and Kalodner C. (2006) Media literacy as a prevention intervention for college women at low- or high-risk for eating disorders. *Body Image* 3: 35–43.

Creed B. (1996) Lesbian bodies – tribades, tomboys and tarts. In E. Grosz and E. Probyn (eds) *Sexy Bodies*, 2nd edn. London: Routledge.

Dokter D. (2000) Arts *Therapies and Clients with Eating Disorders – Fragile Board*. London: Jessica Kingsley.

Eggert J., Levendosky A. and Klump K. (2007) Relationships among attachment styles, personality characteristics, and disordered eating. *International Journal of Eating Disorders* 40(2): 149–55.

Engelin-Maddox R. (2006) Buying a beauty standard or dreaming of a new life? Expectations associated with a new life. *Psychology of Women Quarterly* 30: 258–66.

Everill J., Waller G. and Macdonald W. (1995) Dissociation in bulimia and non-eating disordered women. *International Journal of Eating Disorders* 17(2): 127–34.

Fichter M.M. and Daser C. (1987) Symptomatology, psychosexual development and gender identity in 42 anorexic males. *Psychological Medicine* 17: 409–18.

Feldman M. and Myers I.H. (2007) Eating disorders in diverse lesbian, gay, and bisexual populations. *International Journal of Eating Disorders* 40(3): 218–26.

Friere P. (1970) *Pedagogy of the Oppressed*. New York: Seabury Press.

Gehrman C.A., Hovell M.F., Sallis J.F. and Keating K. (2006) The effects of a physical activity and nutrition on body dissatisfaction, drive for thinness, and weight concerns in pre-adolescents. *Body Image* 3: 345–35.

Ginsberg R.L. and Gray J.J. (2006) The differential depiction of female athletes in judged and non-judged sport magazines. *Body Image* 3: 365–73.

Groesz L.M., Levine M.P. and Murnen S.K. (2002) The effects of experimental presentation of thin media images on body satisfaction: a meta-analytic review. *International Journal of Eating Disorders* 31: 1–16.

Grosz E. and Probyn E. (1996) *Sexy Bodies*. London: Routledge.

Hallings-Pott C., Waller G., Watson D. and Scragg P. (2005) State dissociation in bulimic eating disorders: an experimental study. *International Journal of Eating Disorders* 38(1): 37–41.

Halliwell E. and Dittmar H. (2006) Associations between appearance-related self-discrepancies and young women's and men's affect, body satisfaction, and emotional eating: A comparison of fixed-item and participant-generated self-discrepancies. *Personality and Social Psychology Bulletin* 32: 447–58.

Hatmaker G. (2006) Boys with eating disorders. *Journal of School Nursing* 21(6): 329–31.

Herpertz S., Kielmann R., Wolf A.M., Langkafel M., Senf W. and Hebebrand J. (2003) Does obesity surgery improve psychosocial functioning? A systematic review. *International Journal of Obesity* 27: 1300–14.

Hulley A.J. and Hill A.J. (2001) Eating disorders and health in elite women distance runners. *International Journal of Eating Disorders* 30: 312–7.

James O. (2007) *Affluenza*. London: Vermilion.

Latzer Y., Tzischinsky O. and Azaiza F. (2007) Disordered eating related behaviours among Arab schoolgirls in Israel: an epidemiological study. *International Journal of Eating Disorders* 40(3): 263–70.

Lee H.Y. and Lock J. (2007) Anorexia nervosa in Asian-American adolescents: do they differ from their non-Asian peers? *International Journal of Eating Disorders* 40(3): 227–31.

Levesque M.J. and Vichesky D.R. (2006) Raising the bar on the beautiful: an analysis of the body image concerns of homosexual men. *Body Image* 3: 45–55.

Lipsey Z., Barton S.B., Hulley A. and Hill A.J. (2006) 'After a workout . . .' Beliefs about exercise, eating and appearance in female exercisers with and without eating disorder features. *Psychology of Sport and Exercise* 7: 425–36.

Lowe B., Zipfel S., Buchholz C., Dupont Y., Reas D.L. and Herzog W. (2001) Long-term outcome of anorexia nervosa in a prospective 21-year follow-up study. *Psychological Medicine* 31(5): 881–90.

Lumby C. and Probyn E. (2003) *Remote Control – New Media, New Ethics*. Cambridge: Cambridge University Press.

Lyubomirsky S., Casper R.C. and Sousa L. (2001) What Triggers abnormal eating in bulimic and non-bulimic women? *Psychology of Women Quarterly* 25: 223–32.

Mann W.J. (1988) Laws of desire: has our imagery become over-idealised? In D. Atkins (ed.) Looking Queer: *Body Image and Identity in Lesbian,*

Bisexual, Gay, and Transgender Communities. New York: Harrington Park Press, pp. 345–53.

Morrison M.A., Morrison T.G. and Sager C.L. (2004) Does body satisfaction differ between gay men and lesbian women and heterosexual men and women? A meta-analysis review. *Body Image* 1: 127–38.

National Curriculum (2007) Health promotion and personal and social education. http://www.nc.uk.net and www.gov.uk/en/educationandlearning/schools/ (accessed 2 July 2007).

Noll S.M. and Frederickson B.L. (1998) A mediational model linking self-objectification, body shame and disordered eating. *Psychology of Women Quarterly* 22(4): 623–6.

Norris M.L., Boydell K.M., Pinhas L. and Katzman D.K. (2006) Ana and the internet : a review of pro-anorexia websites. *International Journal of Eating Disorders* 39(6): 443–7.

Orbach S. (1978) *Fat is a Feminist Issue.* Feltham: Hamlyn.

Orbach S. (2006) *Fat is a Feminist Issue.* London: Arrow Books.

Palazzoli M.S. (1978) *Self-starvation.* New York: Jason Aronson.

Probyn E. (2007) Anorexia in the new media. www.wun.ac.uk (accessed 12 November 2007).

Roth A. and Fonagy P. (2006) *What Works For Whom? A critical review of psychotherapy Research*, 2nd edition. London: Guildford Press.

Rothblum E.D. (1994) Lesbians and physical appearance: which model applies? In B. Greene and G.M. Herek (eds) *Lesbian and Gay Psychology: Theory Research and Clinical Applications.* Thousand Oaks, CA: Sage, pp. 84–97.

Schaverin J. (2000) The picture as transactional object in the treatment of anorexia. In D. Dockter (ed.) *Art Therapies and Clients with Eating Disorders.* London: Jessica Kingsley, pp. 31–47.

Schooler D. and Ward L.M. (2006) Average Joes: men's relationships with media, real bodies, and sexuality. *Psychology of Men and Masculinity* 7(1): 27–41.

Slater A. and Tiggemann M. (2002) A test in objectification theory in adolescent girls. *Sex Roles* 46: 343–9.

Sundgot-Borgen J. and Torstveit M.K. (2004) Prevalence of eating disorders in elite athletes is higher than in general populations. *Clinical Journal of Sports Medicine* 14: 25–32.

Swan S. and Andrews B. (2003) The relationship between shame, eating disorders and disclosure in treatment. *British Journal of Clinical Psychology* 42: 367–78.

Szyrynksi V. (1973) Anorexia nervosa and psychotherapy. *American Journal of Psychotherapy* 27: 492–505.

Tiggemann M. and Slater A. (2004) Thin ideals in music television: a source of social comparison and body dissatisfaction. *International Journal of Eating Disorders* 35: 48–58.

Tiggemann M., Martins Y. and Kirkbride A. (2007) Oh to be lean and muscular: body image ideals in gay and heterosexual men. *Psychology of Men and Masculinity* 8(1): 15–24.

Tolman D.L., Impett E.A., Tracy A.J. and Michael A. (2006) Looking good, sounding good: femininity ideology and adolescent girls' mental health. *Psychology of Women Quarterly* 30: 85–95.

Totenbier S.L. and Payne H. (2000) Dance movement therapy. In D. Dokter (ed.) *Arts Therapies and Clients with Eating Disorders – Fragile Board.* London: Jessica Kingsley.

Veale D. (2004) Advances in a cognitive behavioural model of body dysmorphic disorder. *Body Image* 1(1): 113–25.

Wade T.D., Davidson S. and O'Dea J.A. (2003) A preliminary controlled evaluation of a school-based media literacy program and self-esteem program for reducing eating disorder risk factors. *International Journal of Eating Disorders* 33: 371–83.

Weaver A.D. and Byers E.S. (2006) The relationship among body image, body mass index, exercise, and sexual functioning in heterosexual women. *Psychology of Women Quarterly* 30: 333–9.

Wichstrøm L. (2006) Sexual orientation as a risk factor for bulimic symptoms. *International Journal of Eating Disorders* 39(6): 448–53.

Wilksch S.M., Tiggemann M. and Wade T.D. (2006) Impact of interactive school-based media literacy lessons for reducing internalization of media ideals in young adolescent girls and boys. *International Journal of Eating Disorders* 39: 385–93.

Winnicott D.W. (1965) *The Maturational Process and the Facilitating environment.* London: Hogarth Press.

Wykes M. and Gunter B. (2006) *The Media and Body Image.* London: Sage Publications.

Chapter 6

Body image dissatisfaction and psychological challenges

Jo Gilmartin

Introduction

This chapter is concerned with body image dissatisfaction, and initially the associations of obesity, a major challenge in the 21st century. This is a growing public health concern in both developed and underdeveloped countries. Despite the health risks and anxiety spawned in the media, the challenges posed by obesity prevail. The impact of eating disorders has been discussed in Chapter 5 but obesity poses a more robust threat to psychological health and well-being. The focus will be on exploring some of the psychological underpinnings of obesity, issues related to body image disturbance and reviewing the most optimistic interventions for tackling obesity.

The dark underside of body image dissatisfaction and low self-esteem frequently motivates people to pursue cosmetic surgery, a rapidly expanding industry ranging from nose reshaping to face lifts, tummy tucks and breast augmentations. The orientation towards body modification will be considered too. In order to analyse other factors that contribute to the distortion of visible appearance, this chapter explores some specific issues emerging in health care. There is no doubt that the contemporary problem of ageing and visible appearance is indeed challenging, with public attitudes perpetuating negative stereotypes. Above all it is crucial that health professionals empower patients to change the way they think about themselves and work together to achieve body image satisfaction and contented well-being.

Body image dissatisfaction and obesity

Exploring and tackling obesity, with steadily increasing risk factors for poor health and body image disturbance, is in new territory. The National Obesity Forum (2000) in the UK claims that British women are the fattest in Europe, with 23% clinically obese. Men are marginally better at 22.3%. Despite government policy to promote healthier lifestyles (DH 2004), there is a prediction that the majority of people in the UK will be obese by 2030. Obesity in adults is based on the body mass index (BMI) – a BMI of 30 or above is classified as obese, over 35 is known as morbid obesity, and over 40 indicates extreme obesity (DH 2007). However, BMI is calculated according to the Western body. In the context of a more general process of globalisation, obesity is epidemic and is clearly affecting countries such as China and the Gambia. The specific application of a standard BMI might be flawed because of typical differences such as bone density.

The majority of people in the developed world are overweight, including 65% of Americans (Guiliano 2005), and reversing the trend is a major challenge. This huge health concern is being influenced by the fatty fast food industry, busy and inactive lifestyles, poor nutrition and distorted eating behaviour (National Obesity Forum 2000). The magnitude of psychological risks associated with obesity is huge, with the increased likelihood of poor self-esteem, stigmatisation, depression and poor social functioning (DH 2004).

Many white women describe themselves as overweight and express a desire to be thinner believing they are less physically fit than objective assessments reveal (Lynch and Zellner 1999). James (2007: 124) reported that despite local variations the virus driven women, who place high value on appearance, were prone globally to obsessive concern with their weight. Typically, middle-aged women of virus infected China and Singapore aspire to teenage-slim figures. The Muscovite benchmark demonstrates that the Danes are two stones overweight in comparison, giving short shrift to tight fitted short skirts that Muscovites sport. Modern Australian women are influenced by the virus too with 'looking good' high on the agenda.

Women's largeness often fits with the stereotype of woman, the all giving, nurturing, caring, loving, earth mother who excels in caretaking skills (Orbach 2006). There is a tendency for young women in particular to pursue one form of diet or another. Body image dissatisfaction in relation to obesity amongst women is associated with lower self-esteem, depression and disordered eating. The politics of women in visible 'large' bodies is beyond the scope of this chapter but is well articulated by Tischner and Malson (2008). Unsurprisingly, contemporary evidence suggests that men too are dissatisfied with their bodies (Pope et al. 2000). Men also display jarring dissonance to weight issues, falling into two categories, either desiring to lose weight or desiring to gain muscularity (Drewnowski et al. 1995). The majority of gay men idealise a slim body with some expressing a strong desire for muscularity (Yelland and Tiggemann 2003). The increasing value on muscularity with masculinity (Halkitis et al. 2004) among gay men may be an indication of health, which might be significant as the community copes with the impact of HIV/AIDS.

The psychodynamic and feminist perspective

From a psychodynamic and feminist perspective, eating dysfunction is associated with emotional disequilibrium. Orbach (2006: 207) indicates that 'relationships with food symbolise a way of being with the self, for instance, harsh, punitive, inconsistent, depriving, angry, rebellious'. She goes on to suggest that self-dislike is frequently sifted into compulsive eating, to some extent becoming a conveyer belt for the indigestion of uncomfortable emotions (Table 6.1). Binge eating is often followed by self-recrimination and distress (Niego et al. 2007). Arguably, mastery of impulses and excess is a central concern but people frequently measure their dietary achievements by numbers on the scale. There is evidence to suggest that internal order or disorder is a symbol for the emotional, moral and spiritual state of the individual (Bordo 2003). Associations of fat could be mediated by moral qualities, being perceived as 'indicative of laziness, lack of discipline, unwillingness to conform and a poor mastery of the body' (Bordo 2003: 195).

Food provides an oasis of pleasure for many women, with some pointing to feelings of anger, boredom, emptiness, disappointment and loneliness as triggers (Orbach 2006). Eating is used as a tool to cope with emotional turmoil, internal chaos and primal impulses. Food becomes the tranquilliser, suppressing the anxiety that unrecognised feelings raise (Orbach 2006). Compulsive eaters turn to food to meet diverse needs that might arise from unconscious needs and conflicts. Most tend to be out of touch with physiological hunger cues, food permeating with power to provide strength, comfort and personal peace. Contrastingly, female hunger might represent forms of unspeakable desires for sexuality and power. Excess eating might function as a code for the suppression of sexuality (Bordo 2003). Women are only permitted to lust for food when they are pregnant.

Table 6.1 Obesity-domain of psychological experience

Gender	Feeling states/psychological experience	Consequences
Women	Feeling frustrated, feeling unworthy, feeling unattractive, feeling empty, angry, unable to control infantile impulses, internal chaos, despair, feeling isolated, feeling depressed, fear of humiliation, fear of social exclusion, anxiety about sexuality, crushing loneliness, fear of abandonment, feeling stuck, feeling burdened, feeling emotionally hungry	Body dissatisfaction Low self-esteem Target of stereotypes Miserable or defensive about health risks Camouflage make-up and clothing Fantasies about cosmetic surgery Undergoing cosmetic and bariatric surgery
Men	Feeling conscious about bulges, feeling worthless, unaware of blocked emotions, sense of persecution, frustration at loss of potential sexual abilities, disturbed by media ideals, frightened of being controlled, feeling trapped, apathy, envious of fit men, feeling large and powerful, feeling protected	Body disturbance Low or shattered self-esteem Increased gym activity and body building Target of stereotyping Stigmatisation Denial about potential health risks Apathy about exercise Searching web sites about cosmetic surgery Exploring risks and benefits of bariatric surgery

Men's battles

The embarrassing bumps, bulges and large stomachs are often viewed as the enemy and perhaps a poor capacity for self-containment and control of impulses. Contrastingly, Bordo (2003) suggests that the bulging stomachs of mid-nineteenth-century businessmen and politicians were a symbol of bourgeois success. Contemporary associations of obesity are not focused on the accumulations of wealth for men, but perhaps reflect moral or personal inadequacy or lack of will. Men too struggle with attaining a personal grail, food and eating being used to quell anxiety that arises from unconfronted emotional distress (Table 6.1). Adiposity is a major challenge for men because media images of male bodies have become increasingly muscular and V-shaped, emphasising broad shoulders, developed arms and chest muscles, and slim waists (Schooler and Ward 2006: 2).

This mesomorphic (muscular) body type, previously highlighted in Chapter 5, has surged in media portrayals triggering increasing body image dissatisfaction amongst gay and heterosexual men (Tiggemann et al. 2007). Muscularity is tied to cultural meanings, which view men to be powerful, strong, efficacious and physically fit. But at the same time, muscularity has been associated with proletarian status, the insensitive, unintelligent, physically abusive and uncultured body typology (Bordo 2003).

The pursuit of muscularity has become a cultural icon and working out is a glamorised and sexualised activity. Today, it does not signify inferior status, moving away from old associations of muscle with brute. Muscle expresses sexuality, willpower, energy and control of infantile impulses symbolising a positive attitude about one's self-management and appearance. The symbol of pruning and tightening the body might prevent any unwanted or embarrassing emotions to erupt, perhaps encouraging the repression of internal conflicts.

Fatness has functioned in a complex variety of ways for men, some chaotic and stifling. Taken very seriously, it has often meant lack of body adornment, body shame posing a threat to sexual intimacy. Schooler and Ward (2006) suggest that shame may not prevent men from engaging in sexual activity but many withdraw emotionally becoming distant from any potential negative evaluations, thus creating an emotional paralysis that distorts communication flows and a loss of human bondage with their partner. Avoidance coping is a specific consequence of shame (Burgraff 1995), which can lead to denial of the vulnerabilities and anxieties of the physical body.

Pathology, stress and the body

Contrastingly, Ogden et al. (2006) reported that some people attributed their fatness to illness, pregnancy or genetics reflecting a biological approach in regard to cause. The ecological approach to obesity suggests that the contemporary post-agricultural, post-industrial society is 'obesogenic' because it generates too high an equilibrium level of fatness across the whole population. A behavioural model of obesity risk is not specifically determined by genes, but by a dynamic process of interaction between genes and environments (Wardle 2005). The nature of the interplay between divergent responses to food cues might perhaps lead genetically susceptible people to eat more when highly appetising foods are presented.

Yet another proposition put forward by Wardle (2005) is that gene–environment correlations might motivate individuals to seek out palatable foods. Thus as food environments become more liberal, fatness increases in those who are obese (Flegal and Troiano 2000). To some extent this shifts individual responsibility away from personal eating behaviour and lifestyle choices. Recognising 'fatness' feeling states is often a major challenge for some individuals; they are either given little attention or ignored completely. Thus defence mechanisms may unintentionally keep miserable feelings about being fat at bay leading to poor psychological well-being and mental health.

Psychosocial factors can contribute to adiposity. Sarafino (2006) suggests that emotions affect eating patterns. Typically, when people are stressed or experiencing anxiety they tend to eat foods lacking in nutrients with high amounts of unrefined sugar and fats (Dallman et al. 2003) or drink lots of alcohol. Depression too puts people at risk of binge eating (Goodman and Whitaker 2002). Watching television and playing computer games can affect weight gain by decreasing physical activity (Sarafino 2006), which can be a major risk for obese children. Non-surprisingly, many individuals appear to employ a high range of defence mechanisms (Glassman and Hadad 2004) to block out vital contact with the psychological reality. Contrastingly, others feel overwhelmed and bewildered. Between the two extremes there is greater efficacy, when a person will be able to put feelings, motivations and intuition to excellent use (Table 6.2).

In this battle against obesity, we cannot afford to abandon the health threats it poses. Research evidence suggests that obesity is robustly associated with hypertension, heart disease, stroke, diabetes, cancer (Calle et al. 2003; Sarafino 2006) and a poor sense of well-being. Fatness poses disadvantages to a person's health and social relationships in childhood and adulthood (Wadden et al. 2002). Preventing overweight is best encouraged in childhood. However, many current interventions for treating obesity convey negative messages that promote resistance and fail to motivate and sustain public interest.

Table 6.2 Psychological defences and obesity

Psychological defences	Extremely High	Shifting and plummeting	Low
Individual state	'Blocked' 'Shut down' Stuck	'Tuning in' Hopeful	Overwhelmed Greater efficacy

Psychological interventions in prevention and treatment

The control of obesity should not be underestimated, but it is vital not to pathologise people who are obese, perceiving them as bearers of ghastly problems. Crucially, effective interventions bring into focus the uniqueness of each person, and respect and encourage active cooperation for changing behaviour. Tackling obesity, smoking and health inequalities is high on the government agenda. The Wanless (2004) report emphasised the 'fully engaged scenario' aligning the public and government intention for promoting longer, healthier lives and disease prevention, and viewing motivation of the public as a vital feature in controlling obesity. Despite the current severe financial constraints in the health service, there is always freedom for movement, and a possibility for developing a stronger infrastructure to ensure that psychological approaches are utilised on the front line.

Educational strategies for children

Preventing obesity should begin in childhood with the employment of educational strategies to improve body image and strengthen self-esteem. Arguably, in countries such as France education begins with pre-school children. Development models of eating behaviour might be useful for encouraging children to learn and develop healthy food preferences (Ogden 2007). Interventions for children require creativity focusing on the development of healthy lifestyles (DH 2004, 2008) for the family unit. Parents should be taught behavioural modification techniques to control events that preside over their children's eating and exercise patterns. The National Institute for Health and Clinical Excellence (NICE 2006) guidelines on the prevention and management of obesity is a useful resource to employ. Although children are pivotal the whole family must be encouraged to develop behaviour habits that embrace a healthier lifestyle (Chadwick and Croker 2005).

In development terms, intervention programmes to prevent obesity in children require psychosocial support, such as improvements in food available at schools and safe environments for physical activity (Summerbell et al. 2005). Concepts of health promotion are expressed with significance in the National Curriculum (2007), and thus impregnated with cultural meaning and value. This topic is notorious for its difficulties in implementation because children will vary greatly in what they experience and learn, according to their learning style and biography – and hence their capacity to be 'toxic' or 'healthy'. Moreover, in this post-modern era food technology does not appear as sexy or romantic in the national curriculum. Although questions about the ethics of eating have become mainstream, there seems to be a split between the ethics of eating and the ethics associated with teaching about food preparation, healthy nutrition and cooking. If the importance of the former is firmly established in the curriculum, this might help to reduce the penetrating force of globalisation and sharpen the impact of health promotion. To illustrate the importance of such a perspective, Wanless points to state regulatory strategies including regulating information provision, for example, accurate and accessible food labelling, ensuring nutritious school meals, subsidising healthy products (vegetables) and shaping social contexts such as providing school playfields. Evaluating these regulatory strategies for their economic and health impact is also recommended.

Whatever health promotion route is taken, the most powerful intervention (Braet et al. 2003) for treating severely obese children seems to be in-patient, cognitive-behavioural programmes, successful in achieving and maintaining weight loss. School-based interventions should also challenge attitudes and myths about obesity and appearance-related concerns (Rumsey and Harcourt 2004: 167), and prevent bullying, social exclusion and discrimination.

Interventions for adults

Shaw et al.'s (2006) systematic review strongly supports the use of exercise (Figure 6.1) as a weight loss intervention, especially when combined with dietary change. The benefits are well articulated by Ogden (2007 p. 170) including, for example, Box 6.1. Despite the enthusiasm for increasing physical activity (Figure 6.2), reviews shed

---

Box 6.1 Benefits of Exercise

- Reduction in weight and obesity
- Reduction in blood pressure
- Reduction in diabetes
- Reduction in coronary heart disease
- Protection against osteoporosis
- Reduction in depression and anxiety
- Improved self-confidence and self-esteem

Source: Ogden (2007).

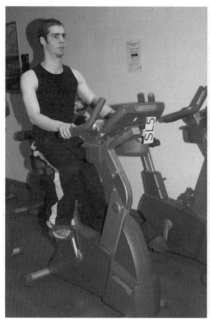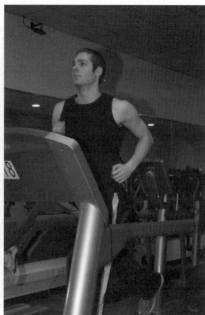

Figure 6.1 and 6.2 Types of gym exercise.

light on different levels of effectiveness. Abraham and Michie (2005: 677) offer a remarkable review linked to Wanless 11 utilising three sources of evidence. The critical sources included a synthesis compiled for the Health Development Agency (Hillsdon et al. 2004); a US systematic review (Kahn et al. 2002) and 18 randomised controlled trials (RCTs) of interventions designed to increase physical activity.

Insights yielded in the Health Development Agency synthesis pointed out that brief advice from a GP, augmented with written information, is possibly effective in producing a modest short-term (6–12 weeks) effect but little evidence of maintenance. Evidence also emphasised that promoting walking or jogging from home rather than using gym facilities was likely to be effective for up to two years. Sustaining physical activity targets by follow-up telephone calls once a week were associated with effectiveness and maintenance. An optimistic view of physical activity intervention for adults aged 50+ emerged in one review, producing mid- to long-term changes in physical activity. Interestingly, the US systematic review (Kahn et al. 2002) displayed strong evidence regarding the effectiveness of community-wide physical activity campaigns (see Box 6.1).

Among other recent reviews of the benefits of exercise, one of the most interesting in Britain is that of Khaw et al. (2008). Their research findings highlighted the importance of combining health behaviours such as non-smoking, physical activity, moderate alcohol intake, and a blood vitamin C greater than 50 mmol/l, indicating fruit and vegetable intake of at least five servings a day. Such a combination predicts a four-fold reduction in the risk of dying over an average period of 11 years for middle aged and older people. They also demonstrate that the risk of death decreases, particularly from cardiovascular disease, as the number of positive health behaviours increases. This evidence is indeed useful to health professionals encouraging modest and achievable lifestyle changes and could have a marked effect on inspiring positive health and well-being. Although this prospective study involved 20,244 women and men aged between 45–79 years with no known cardiovascular disease or cancer, the findings need to be compared to other global populations. Moreover, further analysis of how the combined health behaviours affect quality of life might be helpful in influencing behaviour change.

In addition to the physical benefits of exercise emphasised by Ogden (2007), exercise also results in improved sense of mood and well-being. This is triggered by the release of endorphins, the brain's natural opioids, hence increasing norepinephrine, enhancing mood, self-confidence and self-efficacy, the latter being particularly important for patients with a heavy investment in reducing body mass.

Cognitive behavioural techniques are the most impressive form of intervention for adults too. Chadwick and Croker (2005) suggest a framework that involves educating people about a nutritionally balanced diet by using a variety of cognitive and behavioural techniques to help implement recommendations. Typically, this includes monitoring of food intake with rewards for achieving dietary and physically active goals, a process that might be helpful for achieving modest and sustainable weight loss. Shaw et al.'s (2005) systematic review clearly emphasised the effectiveness of cognitive behavioural therapies in facilitating weight loss. In addition, cognitive models of eating behaviour put forward by Ogden (2007) should be recognised. Cognitions frequently influence the prediction and explanation of eating behaviour and can be utilised too as a means of changing eating behaviour.

Orbach (2006: 343–6) puts forward creative ideas for improving body image, such as experimenting with different exercises on fat/thin and what various body images mean. She goes on to suggest distinguishing body states from emotional states and exploring emotional states in regard to eating patterns. Fatness should not exclude people from 'loving, eating, dancing, running' or living life to the full (Orbach 2006: 252). I suggest that people who take responsibility for weight reduction should try to utilise personal power to shape every aspect

Box 6.2 Body image creative workbook

This is a creative workbook to help you move rapidly towards a positive self-image.

1. What are your usual thoughts and beliefs about body image?
2. What factors influence body image dissatisfaction?
3. Identify any challenges or resistance.
4. Talk to yourself about it and notice how you feel.
5. Search for thoughts that are calming, liberating, reassuring, hopeful or uplifting.
6. Choose more positive thoughts to stabilise that new, uplifted feeling.
7. Choose at least four activities that promote well-being, for example, running, yoga, tai chi, working out in the gym, playing the guitar, writing poetry, singing, dancing, sketching, meditating.
8. Prioritise at least two activities that make you happy in your daily routine.
9. Appreciate and journey every day in this new direction of happiness to increase body image.

of their lives and promote an increasing sense of well-being (Box 6.2). Group therapy can also help people tackle compulsive eating, offering a platform for the exploration of emotional hungers that might be beneficial in breaking the binge cycle.

Recognition is slowly dawning that dance movement therapy (DMT), classified as an art therapy, might also be beneficial. The potential benefits of DMT are vividly described by Meekums (2005), particularly in regard to obesity associated with emotional turmoil and/or distressing life events. This powerful and creative process might enable individuals to shift 'underlying psychological issues that might hinder permanent changes in eating behaviour and body image' (Meekums 2005: 249).

Bariatric surgery

Finally, there is the possibility of using surgery. Morbid obesity (grade III, BMI of 40 and above) is a major contemporary challenge and lifestyle modification without the use of drugs or surgery is perhaps benign and ineffective (Chadwick and Croker 2005). The uptake of bariatric surgery is gaining momentum especially for individuals with 'extensive histories of weight cycling and failed dieting' (Ogden et al.

2006: 289). This invasive procedure is being used more frequently in less severe cases of obesity and raises disturbing questions about the long-term effects of limiting nutritional intake on the growing bodies of adolescents (Santora 2004). Unsurprisingly, the medicalisation of obesity, with its search for solutions exclusively within surgical interventions, serves to distance those affected. The view that people with severe obesity lack insight or cease to be responsible beings rationalises a lack of attention to their poor self-management, and justifies substituting surgical intervention for true, responsible engagement. Obesity and bypass surgery are both on the rise, underscoring the need for a deeper understanding of the psychological causes of obesity.

Nonetheless, Herpertz et al.'s (2003) systematic review highlighted the improved mental health, psychosocial status and employment opportunities following bariatric surgery. The results emphasised considerable improvement in self-esteem and self-confidence in 170 studies reviewed. Ogden et al. (2006) claimed that obesity surgery imposed control, facilitating patient empowerment. These insights were taken further by Niego et al. (2007) who reported that pre-surgical binge eating patterns are more likely to be retained following surgery affecting weight outcomes. Effective management requires a multidimensional treatment approach. Cognitive behavioural therapy has yielded positive results in the treatment of binge eating and might be useful for bariatric surgery candidates to optimise outcomes (Vaidya 2006).

The psychology of body modification

Popular culture is obsessed with appearance and encourages modest to wild fantasies of self-transformation. The rhetoric of choice and self-determination is powerful, eradicating the inequalities of privilege, money and time that disallow the majority from participating (Bordo 2003); but desperation prevails. In some instances, the polysurgical addicts or 'scalpel slaves' pursue a relentless task to reconstruct the body. The dark underside or psychological underpinnings that influence body transformation are triggered by body image dissatisfaction, and low self-esteem. The challenge for health professionals is to help patients explore the profound psychological motives for cosmetic surgery. The conflicts central to breast reduction might in part be a reliance on various forms of splitting mind from body or thought from feeling. The big boob dilemma might be blurred – 'too beautiful', 'too needy', 'too ugly' or 'too sexy'. Drastic action might represent an intensity of feeling that had to be removed, displaying little capacity for containment or careful thinking.

Cosmetic surgery

It is never simple or easy to define the term 'cosmetic' because of its diverse connotations. The representation of 'cosmetic' implies a superficial, trivial meaning, 'only skin deep'. Thus in a culture that views the body as a powerful oracle of expression, as the external representation of the deep inner self, the term 'cosmetic' is fraught with uncertainty (Holliday and Sanchez Taylor 2006). In its original sense, it carries meanings of fake beauty, which could misrepresent a person's motivation to enhance, correct or modify their appearance rather than idealise it. The notion of surgery for the purpose of 'enhancement' is usually labelled as 'cosmetic surgery', mainly facilitated by private medical practice. Holliday and Sanchez Taylor (2006: 187) go on to suggest that the medical establishment downgrades the significance of the latter as 'pandering to the whims of rich, vain women'. Crucially, the outcome for women in terms of increasing self-confidence and optimising well-being is trivialised.

Patients with either visible or invisible appearance related concerns often attend primary care services seeking cosmetic treatments. Some are highly motivated to enhance their appearance whilst others are determined to pursue this contemporary fantasy to its limits fed by modern ideologies of the self. The prevailing emphasis on a positive self-image stimulates the search for the correction of even a small cosmetic imperfection. Almost certainly, the grandiose hope for positive change will increase well-being. Cosmetic surgery is important and healing; some clients are motivated by a desire to improve appearance, others to appease a parent and/or spouse to win love or approval.

Plastic surgery

A technology that was intended to replace malfunctioning parts has gradually generated an industry fuelled by fantasies to transform and sculpt the body into a masterpiece, and correct and defy the mortality and materiality of the body (Bordo 2003). Davis (1995) focuses her interest on the deep psychological anxiety that women experience about their shape, size or perceived body 'defects', claiming that feminists have associated aesthetic surgery with the quest for beauty. However, the women in her study wanted to be 'normal'. In the UK, aesthetic surgery for women experiencing psychological or psychic distress is frequently free and fully approved by the medical establishment, particularly as an intervention to restore 'defective bodies'. This is usually labelled as 'plastic surgery'.

Plastic surgery has become a rapidly expanding industry in both the NHS and the private medical sector, ranging from nose reshaping, ear reshaping, face lifts, tummy tucks and breast augmentations to collagen-plumped lips and liposculpture. Most websites offer a sensational range of surgical and non-surgical treatments with remarkable choices for men and women (www.transforminglives.co.uk/surgery. htm, http://www.harleymedical.co.uk). Genital plastic surgery for women is growing too, encouraging the construction of 'a new frontier' including 'vaginal rejuvenation' and 'labia recasting' (Navarro 2004).

In spite of this expansion, health professionals should be wary of an approach that highlights psychological pain as an argument for plastic surgery. The position taken by Davis (1995) refuting the idea that women are in a quest for beauty is criticised by Holliday and Sanchez Taylor (2006) as a means of denying its importance to women in enhancing status. They go on to suggest that the women interviewed by Davis were seeking free surgery from the state. Similarly, Stone's (1991) appraisal of the medicalised definition of transsexualism stresses that only persons claiming to be in the 'wrong body' and disclosing significant psychological distress are rewarded with medical diagnosis and free surgery. This type of approach does not appear to legitimise truth telling and choice.

Rumsey and Harcourt (2004: 143) point out that a growing number of people who have undergone cosmetic surgery look for plastic surgery in the NHS 'to improve' or 'correct' the outcome of earlier treatments. They go on to suggest that failed cosmetic interventions attract emotional media attention but the evidence base for the psychosocial impact is weak. Cosmetic intervention is an incredibly powerful gift in the beauty industry and might be perceived by potential clients as uncomplicated, with no health risks. Crucially, health professionals need to raise clients' awareness of all implications to elicit genuine consent prior to surgery (Rumsey and Harcourt 2004). It is also critically important to educate people about the psychological features of body-altering procedures and not allow media fantasies to be the determinant of surgery.

Face lifting

The face has huge functional and aesthetic importance. It represents one of the most significant and identifiable aspects of a person's physical being, hence is strongly associated with identity and body image and in everyday life bears significant social and psychological consequences. Improving an aged face and bringing out the beauty that was apparent in youth is crucial to many individuals; surgical rejuvenation of the face has evolved as a very popular procedure. However, despite innovative approaches, improving facial appearance and minimising signs that the surgical procedure has been performed is indeed challenging (Stuzin 2008).

A facelift is the gold standard to correct a sagging, wrinkly neck and jawline (Lewis 2007: 105). Moreover, it has the potential to tighten loose muscle and skin and remove or reposition excess fat to eliminate sagging. There are a variety of different procedures that can be performed, and some helpful suggestions have been offered by Lewis. Patient expectation of face lifting is variable but most view reconstruction surgery as an opportunity for self change and global improvements.

Tattoos and piercing

Procedures such as tattoos and piercing have increased tremendously in popularity and involve a wider range of social class (De Mello 2000). Although frequently recognised as a fashion accessory, deeper psychological meanings are being advanced, such as 'accentuating self-identity' (Atkinson and Young 2001), and 'cultural rebellion and self-definition' (Atkinson 2002). Motivational characteristics are variable and seem to be aligned with a clear sense of purpose (Wohlrab et al. 2007). Nipple and genital piercings appear to be enmeshed with direct sexual stimulation or perhaps emphasise sexuality (Armstrong et al. 2006). Atkinson (2002) reported that the deliberate, painful procedure of tattooing and permanent marking enables abused woman to reclaim a new sense of self.

Men too appear to connect tattoos with their sexuality. A narrative account of a bisexual male, aged 34 years (Holliday and Cairnie 2007: 70), demonstrates that this particular man had acquired and exhibited a large number of tattoos in his youth, signifying 'hard' masculinity (amongst working-class peers) to 'mask' ambiguity about his sexuality. However, when he came out as a bisexual, he underwent skin grafting to erase tattoos on his hands and arms, this process of aesthetic surgery enabling him to realign his body, sexuality and sense of self. We catch a glimpse of how aesthetic surgery can enable a person to experience life in a richer way, with less need to use defence to blank out subjectivity, thus enabling new action schema to be formed, particularly of a relational kind.

Psychological matters of people with visible differences

Abundant psychosocial stressors are linked with being visibly different in a society that places huge weighting on the importance of appearance, beauty and physical attractiveness. Valente (2006) suggests that multiple factors and conditions cause visible differences such as congenital disfigurement, genetic inheritance, growth and development, ageing, accidental trauma, disease and medical or surgical intervention. Throughout this chapter I have emphasised the pathology associated with visible difference in patients grappling with obesity and eating disorders (Chapter 5) including low self-esteem, poor self-image and social isolation. Implicitly, then, the standard paradigm feeds into an extremely negative and deterministic view, which colludes with cultural and media ideals of attractiveness. The prime task of the following sections is to explore the psychological implications of a few specific conditions associated with visible difference, including appropriate interventions to facilitate the enhancement of the existing body.

Cancer patients frequently experience severe psychological distress as a result of being diagnosed with a life-threatening condition, and are frequently exposed to treatments that disrupt or change their appearance. Rumsey and Harcourt (2004: 107) emphasise that some appearance changes are temporary, such as hair loss. Conversely, others are more permanent, for instance, facial asymmetry following the removal of a facial tumour. Other valuable sources (Moyle and Carr 2002; Carr 2003; Lichtenstein et al. 2003) point to lipoatrophy syndrome which is a risk for HIV patients treated with highly active antiretroviral therapy (Patella et al. 1988) to control HIV infection. This syndrome has a marked impact on altered appearance; for example, patients might develop carinofacial lipoatrophy, limb lipoatrophy, 'double chin' and 'buffalo hump'. This can trigger emotional distress, labelling and social isolation.

Hair loss

Hair loss caused by cancer treatment represents a symbolic loss of self, a visible illustration of cancer diagnosis (Pickar-Holley 1995; Richer and Ezer 2002; Rosman 2004), imprisonment in terrifying loneliness and the personal danger of a bare head. The complete process might be regarded as an 'involuntary downward spiral', in which self-image is radically or gradually undermined. Reactions and attitudes from family members or society may vary, and include stigmatisation, avoidance or over-protectiveness. At the very least patients can try to disguise or contain the perceived worst aspects of appearance by using wigs. The effect of camouflage could be theoretically embracing to patients who value the wig aesthetic but there may be a contrasting dislike by patients who perceive wigs to be unnatural (Williams 1999) or disguising. Nonetheless, the threshold of body image disturbance might attain an adjustment moving to further stability as hair starts to re-grow.

On the other hand, hair transplants by men are becoming more common. This procedure is carried out under local anaesthetic, facilitating the transplantation of 1,000 to 4,000 follicles per session. The process might involve three or four sessions depending on idiosyncratic aspirations. Aesthetic surgery can help bodies to be realigned with the perceived self, especially when the self is experiencing life changes. Thus the notion of identity might be influential in the decision making process about aesthetic surgery. Holliday and Cairnie (2007: 66) offer an interesting account of a heterosexual male, aged 47 years, middle-class, divorced with three children, who began a relationship with a woman 20 years his junior (after his divorce), and then proceeded to obtain a hair transplant. This brought about positive changes to his identity with significant effects on body and psychological health. Despite the small sample size, this success story is particularly encouraging for men wrestling with the body aesthetic.

Facial disfigurement

Facial disfigurement has received much research interest because of the unique functional importance of the face. Significantly, patients with head and neck cancer frequently experience facial asymmetry (Valente 2006), loss or impairment of speech and swallowing, leaving some prone to psychological and social problems (Partridge and Rumsey 2003). It is noteworthy that some patients feel stigmatised, receive negative remarks, and are confronted with naked stares, avoidance, and unpleasant behaviour from others (Clarke 1999). Taken to an extreme, some individuals may describe subjective feelings of ugliness associated with the physical defect leading to body dysmorphic disorder. A crucial factor in understanding the psychological distress is the severity of the facial disfigurement and social self-efficacy moderators (Brill et al. 2006; Hagedoorn and Molleman 2006).

The nature of the distress process can be constructed as a dialectical interplay between facial disfigurement induced impairment and malignant social psychology, which is probably universal to all individuals who receive intervention for head, face and neck cancer.

The contributions made by the treatment intervention impairment will vary from one person to another; and the content of the malignant social psychology will also range from staring and stigmatisation, to avoidance or stereotypical comments. In most instances the severity of the disfigurement will determine different psychological states; a person may go through a fairly rapid decline and feel depressed, then attain a sense of equilibrium, stay on a plateau, attain further stability, and so on. Hagedoorn and Molleman (2006: 646) reported that when social self-efficacy was high, regardless of the degree of facial disfigurement, patients perceived little social isolation.

Another factor to consider is the psychological impact of facial laceration from patients presenting themselves at an emergency department. A study undertaken by Tebble et al. (2006) reported that patients with larger scars (4 cm or greater) had significantly higher anxiety and self-consciousness scores than patients with smaller scars. This was apparent after both one week and six months. Patients who fell in the assault or accident category had higher scores at one week and six months in comparison to the participants whose injuries were sports related. They also reported that the psychological consequence of facial laceration was influenced by psychosocial factors. Typically, patients who were married or lived with a partner had a significantly lower general self-consciousness at both time points (Tebble et al. 2006: 524). This might infer that individuals in long-term relationships are less conscious of visible appearance.

Aesthetic surgery for facial disfigurement

Aesthetic surgery might be an option for some patients with self-enhancement aspiration following facial disfigurement or scarring. The notion of self-enhancement is eloquently portrayed by Holliday and Sanchez Taylor (2006: 189), the central idea being that enhancement does not suggest body transformation but working 'with' the body the patient already has – 'the (self) improvement of the existing body – its enhancement as opposed to the promise of a different body'. It is not surprising that the decision making process about aesthetic surgery requires careful consideration. Holliday and Cairnie (2007) report a striking narrative of a 52-year-old police officer, who received facial injury when attacked on duty with a knife. He believed that his scar brought him negative attention and limited promotional opportunities. Ten years after the injury, and encouraged by his wife, he successfully underwent a rinoplasty, cheek reconstruction and series of scar revision procedures. The aesthetic surgery seemed to have significant positive outcomes for this man in terms of 'self-identity' and 'social identity'. Indeed, although subtle messages about body image are conferred by others, to have an identity is to know who one is, both in feeling and cognition.

Self-efficacy and social integration

Newell (2000) offers a major contribution towards encouraging patients with disfigurement to confront psychosocial difficulties by increasing self-efficacy and social integration. He points to cognitive behavioural therapy as a useful intervention, enabling patients to form effective coping strategies for successful body image integration. Brill et al. (2006) put forward another significant framework for the anticipation and management of body image issues in facial transplantation. They go on to suggest that cognitive behavioural approaches are indeed powerful, allowing vulnerable patients to explore anxiety, depression, functional difficulties and social avoidance.

Clearly health professionals need to employ sensitive language to communicate with patients. For example, 'the graft' should always be referred to as 'your face' and the patients encouraged to use verbal utterances such as 'my face' (Brill et al. 2006: 11). The rehabilitative process should include education in social skills and assertion training too, thus enabling individuals following disfigurement to take the lead in dialogue, avoid colluding with social norms and move from the shadow to the limelight gracefully. This can be helpful at promoting social integration and reducing heightened self-consciousness and social anxiety (Rumsey and Harcourt 2004).

It is often possible to discover a person's attitude towards increasing positive well-being. Some might have a real aptitude for meditation/ yoga, or singing or walking in nature, or playing a musical instrument. It is vital to establish routes for individuals to relax and encourage the utilisation of 'brain gym' techniques that enhance the release of anxiety, negative thoughts or troublesome feelings, hence promoting inner peace and a greater sense of self.

Ageing and visible appearance

The rapid growth in the ageing population throughout the world has led to a dramatic increase in awareness of body image dissatisfaction and outward appearance. Rumsey and Harcourt (2004: 84) point to a number of factors associated with body image disturbance including hair loss and colour, skin sagging, pronounced wrinkles, visible changes to the chin, earlobes and nose. The anxieties around ageing centre too on changing chronic conditions such as the impact of arthritis and obesity on joints, the powerlessness of mobility, postural and elimination challenges, and the decline in sexual attractiveness. This is sometimes compounded by the extreme vulnerability associated with the use of unwelcome visible aids (Tiggemann 2004).

Moreover, the frailty associated with ageing and changing physical appearance can provoke a 'loss of self' and a poor self-image. It is likely that a range of powerful and contradictory emotions might be aroused in patients: fear, anxiety, anger, disgust, envy and sexual desire. Of course the meaning and priority afforded to body image is often downplayed in an older adult context, particularly where defence processes are entrenched, and so neglecting the subtle tasks of psychological care. There are varies tactics that can be employed for putting body image issues at a distance, including stereotyping and dehumanising labels.

Male sexuality

Male sexual performance in regard to ageing has become medicalised since the 1980s with a major focus on understanding erectile problems (Tiefer 1986). Gott (2005) also suggests that urologists emphasise the vascular and physiological factors associated with impotence, ignoring psychological factors. The conceptual and medical interest in understanding erectile dysfunction, coupled with media attention, triggered the huge pharmaceutical and commercial success of Viagra (Gott 2005: 35). This impacted on individual beliefs and values with respect to 'social worth' and 'sexual energy', encouraging 'pill pushing' as a cure for the masculine struggle. The contemporary culture too, technologically and cosmetically armed, seems bent on defying ageing, insisting on the 'law of lust' against the spiritual and psychological will to gain equilibrium. Continuing historical power and pervasiveness of certain cultural images and ideology leave men (and women too) feeling vulnerable.

Gradually over the last century, but accelerating into the 21st century, the status of sexuality, body image and ageing has been enhanced. These developments attempt to transcend negative stereotyping, dismantle prejudice and embrace a deeper and richer understanding of later life sexuality. Gott (2005) attempts to sexualise old age with intent, recognising individual need, human rights and freedom. Crucially, this liberating paradigm needs to be cemented in healthcare systems, the process of care acknowledging gender difference and need, enabling a person to become more aware and more in touch with sexual desire and fulfilment. Although Gott advances ideas to revolutionise body image and ageing, some have been commonplace for some time. Therefore it is vital that health practitioners try to make dynamic sense of the current beauty and aesthetic landscape and interpret its significance for enhancing body image in older women and men.

Conclusion

- The challenges posed by obesity in terms of body image dissatisfaction, and the consequences for men and women, are examined.
- The psychodynamic and feminist perspective of eating dysfunction is explored in relation to emotional turmoil.
- Psychosocial factors that contribute to obesity are considered, including stress, depression and watching television.
- Research evidence and policy directives regarding effective psychological and educational interventions in the prevention and treatment of obesity for both children and adults are emphasised.
- The usefulness of bariatric surgery as an intervention is also briefly examined.
- Psychological problems of people with visible difference (for example, hair loss, facial disfigurement and the ageing process) point to normative discontent.
- The major psychological problems experienced by people with appearance related concerns relate to low or shattered self-esteem, the impact appearance has on others, negative self-perceptions and fear of stereotyping and stigmatisation.
- Drawing on research evidence the dilemmas and benefits of contemporary interventions to enhance body image such as cosmetic and plastic surgery are explored, particularly in relation to self-enhancement.
- Despite the wide range of research methodologies that have been utilised, there is scope for use of prospective and longitudinal research especially in relation to the risks and benefits of aesthetic surgery.

References

Abraham C. and Michie S. (2005) Contributing to public health policy and practice. *The Psychologist* 18: 11.

Armstrong M.L., Caliendo C. and Roberts A.E. (2006) Genital piercings: what is known and what genital piercings tell us. *Urologic Nursing* 26: 173–80.

Atkinson M. (2002) Pretty in ink: conformity, resistance, and negotiation in women's tattooing. *Sex Roles* 47: 219–35.

Atkinson M. and Young K. (2001) Flesh journey: neo primitives and the contemporary rediscovery of radical body modification. *Deviant Behaviour* 22: 117–46.

Brill S.E., Clarke A., Veal D.M. and Butler P.E.M. (2006) Psychological management and body image issues in facial transplantation. *Body Image* 3: 1–15.

Bordo S. (2003) *Unbearable Weight. Feminism, Western Culture, and the Body*. London: University of California Press.

Braet C., Tanghe A., De Bode P., Franckx H. and Van Winckel M. (2003) Impatient treatment of obese children. *European Journal of Pediatrics* 162: 391–6.

Burgraff S.A. (1995) Coping styles related to shame-and-guilt proneness. Poster presentation at the annual meeting of the Eastern Psychological Association, Boston. In Schooler D. and Ward L.M. (2006). Average Joes: men's relationships with media, real bodies, and sexuality. *Psychology of Men and Masculinity* 7(1): 27–41.

Calle E.E., Rodriguez C., Walker-Thurmond K. and Thun M.J. (2003) Overweight, obesity, and morality from cancer in a prospective studies cohort of US adults. *New England Journal of Medicine* 57: 1–11.

Carr A. (2003) HIV lipodystrophy: risk factors, pathogenesis, diagnosis and management. *Aids* 17(Suppl. 1): S141–8.

Chadwick P. and Croker H. (2005) Obesity management. *The Psychologist* 18(4): 220–3.

Clarke A. (1999) Psychosocial aspects of facial disfigurement: problem management and the role of a lay-led organisation. *Psychology, Health and Medicine* 4(2): 127–42.

Cosmetic Surgery (2007) www.transforminglives.co.uk/surgery.htm (accesssed 18 October 2007) Cosmetic Surgery http://www.harleymedical.co.uk (accessed 18 October 2007).

Dallman M.F., Pecoraro N., Akana S.F., La Fleur S.E., Gomez F., Houshayer H. et al. (2003) Chronic stress and obesity: a new view of 'comfort food'. *Proceedings of the National Academy of Sciences* 100: 11696–701.

Davis K. (1995) *Reshaping the Female Body: The Dilemma of Cosmetic Surgery*. London: Routldedge.

De Mello M. (2000) Bodies of inscriptions: a cultural history of the modern tattoo community. Durham: Duke University Press.

Department of Health (DH) (2004) Initiatives to promote healthier lifestyles. http://www.dh/gov.uk (accessed 2 July 2007).

Department of Health (2008) Healthy Weight, Healthy Lives, a Cross-Government Strategy for England. http://www.dh/gov.uk (accessed 20 February 2008).

Drewnowski A., Kurth C.L. and Krahn D.D. (1995) Effects of body image on dieting, exercise, and anabolic steroid use in adolescent males. *International Journal of Eating Disorders* 17: 381–6.

Flegal K.M. and Troiano R.P. (2000) Changes in the distribution of body mass index of adults and children in the US population. *International Journal of Obesity* 24: 807–18.

Glassman W.E. and Hadad M. (2004) *Approaches to Psychology*, 4th edition. Maidenhead: Open University Press.

Goodman E. and Whitaker R.C. (2002) A prospective study of the role of depression in the development and persistence of adolescent obesity. *Pediatrics* 109: 497–504.

Gott M. (2005) *Sexuality, Sexual Health and Ageing*. Maidenhead: Open University Press.

Guiliano M. (2005) *French Women Don't Get Fat*. London: Chatto and Windus.

Hagedoorn M. and Molleman E. (2006) Facial disfigurement in patients with head and neck cancer: the role of social self-efficacy. *Health Psychology* 25(5): 643–7.

Halkitis P.N., Green K.A. and Wilton L. (2004) Masculinity, body image, and sexual behaviour in HIV-seropositive gay men: a two phase formative behavioural investigation using the Internet. *International Journal of Men's Health* 3: 27–42.

Herpertz S., Kielmann R., Wolf A.M., Langkafel M., Senf W. and Hebebrand J. (2003) Does obesity surgery improve psychosocial functioning? A systematic review. *International Journal of Obesity* 27: 1300–14.

Hillsdon M., Foster C., Naidoo B. and Crombie H. (2004) A review of the evidence on the effectiveness of public health intervention for increasing physical activity among adults: a review of reviews. London: Health Development Agency.

Holliday R. and Cairnie A. (2007) Man made plastic. Investigating men's consumption of aesthetic surgery. *Journal of Consumer Culture* 7(1): 57–78.

Holliday R. and Sanchez Taylor J. (2006) Aesthetic surgery as false beauty. *Feminist Theory* 7(2): 179–218.

James O. (2007) *Affluenza*. London: Vermilion.

Kahn E.B., Ramsey L.T., Brownson R. et al. (2002) The effectiveness of interventions to increase physical activity. *American Journal of Preventive Medicine* 22: 73–105.

Khaw K.T., Wareham N., Bingham S., Welch A., Luben R. and Day N. (2008) Combined impact of health behaviours and mortality in men and women: the EPIC-Norfolk Prospective Population Study. *PloS Medicine* 5(1): e12.

Lewis W. (2007) *Plastic Makes Perfect. The complete cosmetic beauty guide*. London: Orion Publishing Group.

Lichtenstein K.A., Delaney K.M., Armon C., Ward D.J., Moorman A.C., Wood K.C. et al. (2003) Incidence of and risk factors for lipoatrophy (abnormal fat loss) in ambulatory HIV-1-infected patients. *Journal of Acquired Immune Deficiency Syndrome* 32: 48–56.

Lynch S.M. and Zellner D.A. (1999) Figure preference in two generations of men: the use of figure drawings illustrating differences in muscle mass. *Sex Roles* 40: 833–43.

Meekums B. (2005) Responding to the embodiment of distress in individuals defined as obese: implications for research. *Counselling and Psychotherapy Research* 5(3): 246–55.

Moyle G. and Carr A. (2002) HIV-associated lipodystrophy, metabolic complications, and antiretroviral toxicities. *HIV Clinical Trials* 3: 89–98.

Navarro M. (2004) The most private of makeovers. *The New York Times, Sunday Styles* November 28: 1.

Newell R. (2000) *Body Image and Disfigurement Care*. London: Routledge.

National Curriculum (2007) Health promotion and personal and social education. http://www.nc.uk.net and www.gov.uk/en/educationandlearning/schools/ (accessed 2 July 2007).

National Institute for Health and Clinical Excellence (NICE) (2006) *Guidelines on the Prevention of Obesity*. Available online at www.nice.org.uk (accessed 18 July 2007).

National Obesity Forum (2000) The growing impact of obesity on patients in the NHS. http://nationalobesityforum.org.uk (accessed 30 June 2007).

Niego S.H., Kofman M.D., Weiss J.J. and Geliebter (2007) Binge eating in the bariatric surgery population: a review of the literature. *International Journal of Eating Disorders* 40(4): 349–59.

Ogden J. (2007) *Health Psychology*. Maidenhead: Open University Press.

Ogden J., Clementi C. and Aylwin S. (2006) The impact of obesity surgery and the paradox of control: a qualitative study. *Psychology and Health* 21(2): 273–93.

Orbach S. (2006) *Fat is a Feminist Issue*. London: Arrow Books.

Patella F.J. Jr, Delaney K.M., Moorman A.C., Loveless M.O., Fuhrer J., Satten G.A. et al. (1988) Declining morbidity and mortality among patients with advanced human immunodeficiency virus infection. HIV Outpatient Study Investigation. *New England Journal of Medicine* 338: 853–60.

Partridge J. and Rumsey N. (2003) Skin scarring: new insights may make adjustments easier. *British Medical Journal* 326: 765.

Pickar-Holley S. (1995) The symptom experience of alopecia. *Seminars in Oncology Nursing* 11(4): 235–8.

Pope H.G., Phillips K.A. and Olivardia R. (2000) The Adonis complex: the secret crisis of male body obsession. New York: The Free Press.

Richer M. and Ezer H. (2002) Living in it, living with it and moving on: dimensions of meaning during chemotherapy. *Oncology Nursing Forum* 29(1): 113–19.

Rosman S. (2004) Cancer and stigma: experience of patients with chemotherapy induced alopecia. *Patient Education and Counselling* 52: 333–9.

Rumsey N. and Harcourt D. (2004) *The Psychology of Appearance.* Maidenhead: Open University Press.

Santora M. (2004) Beyond baby fat. *The New York Times, The Metro Section* November 26: B1.

Sarafino E.P. (2006) *Health Psychology. Biopsychosocial Interactions*, 5th ed. New York: John Wiley & Sons.

Schooler D. and Ward L.M. (2006) Average Joes: men's relationships with media, real bodies, and sexuality. *Psychology of Men and Masculinity* 7(1): 27–41.

Shaw K., Gennat H., O'Rourke P. and Del Mar C. (2006) Exercise for overweight or obesity. *Cochrane Database of Systematic Reviews* 2007 Issue 2.

Stone S. (1991) The Empire strikes back: a posttranssexual manifesto. In K. Straub and J. Epstein (eds) *Body Guards: The Cultural Politics of Gender Ambiguity.* New York: Routledge, pp. 280–304.

Stuzin J.M. (2008) Face lifting. *Journal of the American Society of Plastic and Reconstructive Surgery* 121(IS): 1–19.

Summerbell C.D., Waters E., Edmunds L.D., Kelly S., Brown T. and Campbell K.J. (2005) Interventions for preventing obesity in children. *Cochrane Database of Systematic Reviews* 2007 Issue 2.

Tebble N.J., Adams R., Thomas D.W. and Price P. (2006) Anxiety and self-consciousness in patients with facial lacerations one week and six months later. *British Journal of Oral and Maxillofacial Surgery* 44: 520–5.

Tiggemann M. (2004) Body image across the adult lifespan: stability and change. *Body Image* 1: 29–41.

Tiggemann M., Martins Y. and Kirkbride A. (2007) Oh to be lean and muscular: body image ideals in gay and heterosexual men. *Psychology of Men and Masculinity* 8(1): 15–24.

Tiefer L. (1986) In pursuit of the perfect: the medicalization of male sexuality. *American Behavioural Scientist* 29: 579–99.

Tischner I. and Malson H. (2008) Exploring the politics of women's in/visible 'large' bodies. *Feminism and Psychology* 18(2): 260–7.

Vaidya V. (2006) Cognitive behavioural therapy of binge eating disorder. *Advanced Psychosomatic Medicine* 27: 86–93.

Valente S.M. (2006) Visual disfigurement and depression. *Plastic Surgical Nursing* 24(4): 140–8.

Wadden T.A., Brownell K.D. and Foster G.D. (2002) Obesity: responding to the global epidemic. *Journal of Consulting and Clinical Psychology* 70: 510–25.

Wanless D. (2004) *Securing Good Health for the Whole Population.* http:// www.dh/gov.uk (accessed 2 July 2007).

Wardle J. (2005) The triple whammy. *The Psychologist* 18(4): 16–19.

Williams J. (1999) A narrative study of chemotherapy induced alopecia. *Oncology Nursing Forum* 26(9): 1463–8.

Wohlrab S., Stahl J. and Kappeler P.M. (2007) Modifying the body: motivations for getting tattooed and pierced. *Body Image* 4: 87–95.

Yelland C. and Tiggemann M. (2003) Muscularity and the gay ideal: body dissatisfaction and disordered eating in homosexual men. *Eating Behaviour* 4: 107–16.

Chapter 7

Communication and mental health

Pauline Phillips

Introduction

This chapter is about mental health and about the importance of communication in the development and maintenance of mental health. It focuses on two psychological approaches to the development of mental health and mental illness, and these have been chosen because each, despite their many differences, has implications for how we communicate with our patients and the effects this may have on their mental health.

The chapter is, however, targeted at all healthcare practitioners and not primarily at those working specifically in mental health settings. This is because serious physical ill health, pain, accidents, disability and disease threaten mental health (Freshwater 2006). Skilled communication, which is at the heart of psychological care, is often lacking, despite its clearly demonstrated mental and physical benefits and seen as the cherry on the icing on the cake of healthcare, rather than a fundamental aspect of assessment and treatment which facilitates recovery and rehabilitation and promotes mental health.

Indeed it can be argued that psychological care, as distinct from physical treatment, is not even in abundance in the mental health field, where it might be most expected. Whittington and McLaughlin (2000) found that on three acute admission wards in Northern Ireland, only 42% of the nurses' day was spent communicating with patients and a mere 6.75% of their time was spent in any potentially therapeutic endeavour. Bee et al. (2006) reported similar findings from their investigation into nursing activity in acute inpatient mental healthcare settings, which found that the majority of the patient-staff interaction was with unqualified staff and that little structured therapeutic care was provided.

I am not, however, suggesting that health practitioners of any discipline deliberately or maliciously neglect the mental health of their clients. It is understandable to want to protect yourself from the perceived stresses and demands of addressing mental health needs, especially if these are poorly understood. Nevertheless, ignoring the mental health needs of patients or simply not understanding and responding to them in the short term can lead to greater problems for patients. This will eventually make further demands on the time of healthcare professionals. Davis and Fallowfield (1991) have explained at length how poor communication leads to a reluctance by the patient to freely express their individual problems or concerns and how this can lead to dissatisfaction, poor compliance and even inaccurate diagnosis. Anxiety and depression are more likely, rehabilitation may be compromised and the necessary psychological adjustment and adaptation to the health problem made more difficult.

My aim, therefore, is to offer all healthcare practitioners two psychological models of mental health which can help them understand, from a theoretical perspective, the importance of their communication with clients. The psychological approaches to mental health I discuss in this chapter, are the *psychoanalytic* and the *cognitive-behavioural* approaches. Both of these approaches have a breadth and depth of theories and concepts which are well described and explained elsewhere, however, there are within them elements which can enhance our understanding of the nature and consequences of good communication in healthcare.

Mental health

The World Health Organization has defined *mental health* as 'a state of well-being in which the individual realizes his or her own abilities, can cope with the normal stresses of life, can work productively and fruitfully, and is able to make a contribution to his or her own community' (WHO, 2001: 1).

Western psychiatry makes the assumption that its theories and diagnoses are valid across cultures. Yet 'a state of well-being', demonstrated, according to this definition, by certain behaviours, necessitates a culture and environment in which the realisation of one's own abilities is possible, encouraged and facilitated. Resources need to be accessible to deal with whatever are considered 'the normal stresses of life', which will vary from culture to culture, and productive and fruitful work must be available. Such a definition is based on the premise that the perception of mental health and mental illness is highly dependent on the values and politics of the culture and society in which people live. 'The politics of the external world enters into the mind of the individual' (Frosh: 999: 38). The potential impact on the body image and self-esteem of individuals of current media ideals and values, and the stereotypes generated, is an example of this and is discussed at length in Chapter 5. Healthcare settings have their own values, culture and politics, determined partly by those of the wider society, partly by the individuals who work in those settings and partly by the nature of the work and its effect on those individuals. As healthcare professionals, we become part of the external world of our patients, often when they are at their most mentally vulnerable and dealing with far more than the 'normal stresses of life'. Therefore, what is spoken about and how, and perhaps more significantly, what is *not* spoken of, and the messages this conveys can have a profound effect on our patients' physical and mental health and on their recovery and rehabilitation.

Nicholls (2003: 27), points out that 'common psychological reactions to illness and injury include shock and even post-traumatic stress, confusion and distress, loss of self-worth, lowered personal control and a collapse into dependency'.

Some patients, of course, may need more specialised psychological care for these problems and an awareness of the need for a referral to other services is part of giving good mental healthcare. However, we do not need to be trained psychologists or counsellors to be able to listen to our patients, to understand their perceptions and to respond therapeutically. Our own attitudes to health, illness, disease and death will influence how we care for our patients. Our own values, those of the culture in which we work and live, and our own inner resources will affect how we communicate with them.

It is estimated that in the UK, mental illness is the primary cause of 40% of disability and that a third of people consulting their general practitioner have mental health problems, which occupy a third of the GPs' time (LSE 2006). Each of the different approaches to psychology has its own theories about mental illness, about how and why it occurs. We refer to mental and physical illness as separate domains, and there are separate centres for treatment, often employing healthcare practitioners with differing and distinct qualifications and skills. It is difficult not to write and talk about the physical and the mental domains as separate entities. Nevertheless it is true that for every 'mental' experience or phenomenon, a physiological process is occurring. It is equally true that those experiences we label physiological or biological also involve mental processes and effects. Psychologists might be more likely to refer to 'psychological disturbance' or 'psychopathology' than mental illness, to avoid the implication that such a condition is solely attributable to a sickness that can be medically investigated, diagnosed and physically treated. However, there are many psychologically disabling conditions which have been found to have specific physical origins, for example hypothyroidism, the symptoms of which include depressed mood and memory impairment (Rinomhota and Marshall 2000). Nevertheless, there is, however, a growing awareness of the multiple social, psychological and biological factors which affect the mental health of individuals and of society (WHO 2005) and an acknowledgement of the interaction between physical and mental health.

A psychodynamic approach to mental health

This approach to mental health is derived from theories of psychoanalysis and at its heart, indeed what makes it distinct from other perspectives, is the notion of the unconscious. Psychoanalytic theories have been expanded and revised since they were first developed by Freud and discussion of the many different models and schools of psychoanalysis is beyond the scope of this chapter. However, the following principles are agreed. I would like to explain how each of these has relevance in general health care.

Our feelings, thoughts and behaviour are influenced by processes of which we are not totally aware

The central tenet of the psychodynamic approach is the notion of the unconscious and how it influences us. The idea of unconscious mental processes had long been considered and written about, for centuries before psychoanalysis (Ellenberger 1970), but Freud was the one of the first to study it in detail and to consider how it influenced our every day functioning. It can be really helpful to realise that we might be driven by processes which are out of our awareness, when we are puzzled and frustrated by our own patterns of behaviour and relationships as well as those of our patients.

Freud concluded that the unconscious followed different rules from those processes which we are aware of. In unconscious mental activity, images and ideas become blended, and any idea or object, and the emotional world these represent, can be symbolised by any other idea or object. Thus the unconscious contains hidden meaning. Although many of Freud's ideas about the unconscious have not been supported by empirical evidence, modern cognitive psychology has clearly demonstrated the existence of unconscious processes. There is also support for Freud's argument that unconscious processes are not limited by those of conscious intention and logic (Power 2000). If we can bear in mind that the vulnerability and uncertainty that illness brings can trigger many unconscious processes and associations, we may be less perplexed and more understanding when patients have seemingly irrational reactions to their illness and treatment.

As adults, the pattern of our earliest relationships, and the emotions and behaviours associated with them may be activated and intensified with those from whom we expect help and care

Our patients are probably unaware (unconscious) of how much their reactions to what is happening to them may have been influenced by childhood experiences. For example, what does it mean to be brave or strong, to be weak or helpless? Is it acceptable to be angry, upset, devastated, terrified or are stoicism, passive cooperation and gratitude the qualities that are valued and that healthcare professionals expect and approve of, in themselves and in others? Freud (1923) argued that the family was the mediating agency through which the values of society were transmitted to individuals. The internalisation of these values he called the superego which is an aspect of the mind which has the capacity to punish the individual, through guilt, when there is a perceived failure to uphold these values. The point is well made in Chapter 3 that autonomy and independence are so highly valued in British society that their loss, through illness or injury, especially when this is long term, may make the feelings associated with such loss more intense and the adjustment to it more difficult.

It had been noticed, long before Freud, that people tend to develop intense feelings, both positive and negative, towards those in whom they regularly confide. It is to Freud's eternal credit that when a female patient did make a physical advance towards him, throwing her arms around him as she came out of the hypnosis which he used at that time, he neither took advantage of this nor abandoned his patient in fright as Breuer, one of his colleagues, had done in similar circumstances. He was able to consider what was happening and how it would be best dealt with (Freud 1925). The imbalance of power was acknowledged and the concept of transference developed and used to better understand the patient. *Transference* refers to the way in which the feelings, wishes and actions of the patient in relation to the nurse, therapist or counsellor may be unconsciously influenced, coloured or distorted by childhood experiences, especially with parents. Freud was the first person to systematically investigate its psychological and therapeutic significance (Freud 1958).

As healthcare professionals, we are part of a huge organisation whose purpose is to promote and advise on health and to treat and care for sick people. Even if our patients are exclusively adults, we represent nurturing, care and a certain degree of authority, as parents usually do to their children. It is therefore not surprising that our patients sometimes develop strong feelings about us. The relationships our patients had with their parents or early carers can unconsciously be transferred to someone in adult life who looks after them. This is recognised by the Nursing and Midwifery Council (NMC 2002: 11) who refer to the need for 'in-depth understanding of relationship issues and the processes whereby a client transfers experiences and expectations from the past onto the practitioner'.

Anderson and Miranda (2000) investigated this process when they asked those taking part in their study for information about the most significant people in their childhood, usually their parents. They were then given a description of another person with some of the specific attributes of these significant people, as they had recounted them. They were later asked to recall this description. The participants would remember the characteristics of this new person but they tended to add extra ones, not included in the description, which they had earlier also used to describe their parents. So, in this experimental situation, when thinking about a new person with similarities to a parent, a mental representation of the parental figure was triggered and 'transferred' to the new person. This offers some support for the existence of the real life phenomenon in which the 'here and now' of a relationship is distorted; in healthcare, the emotionally laden mental representations of care and authority built up in childhood can be unconsciously triggered in the present (Anderson and Miranda 2000). See Box 7.1.

The messages we convey, therefore, in the healthcare setting, about what may and may not be spoken of, about what will be heard and responded to and what will be blocked, can have a significant impact on how our patients process their experiences of injury, disease and loss and ultimately on their mental health.

If we sense that our feelings and impulses may be overwhelmingly painful or unacceptable to ourselves and/or others, we use strategies, called mental defence mechanisms, to keep them out of awareness

Children receive messages sometimes explicitly and sometimes very subtly, from parents and from the wider society about what is considered 'normal' and acceptable, what is unacceptable, weak or wicked

Box 7.1 Example of transference and the past repeating in the present

John's father had severe alcohol problems and had been unable to provide for his family emotionally or financially because of this. John often had to help his mother cope with his father's disruptive behaviour. As the eldest in the family, John had started earning money, doing paper rounds and other jobs as soon as he was able, to help support the family. By early adulthood he had developed a very successful business and become the family's main support, helping everyone with money and advice.

When he was 27 he was seriously injured in a road traffic accident which left him in a coma for several weeks and afterwards in need of nursing care, at first in hospital and then at home, for over a year. He resisted, as much as possible, the nurses' attempts to help him, was very reluctant to take painkillers, and embarked on his physical rehabilitation with the most determination the physiotherapist had ever seen.

Discussion point

According to the psychodynamic approach, why might John have found it so difficult to accept the help and pain relief that was available? What was he transferring from the past to the present?

(As a child he had cut himself off from any feelings of vulnerability and helplessness, in response to his circumstances. When such feelings, long buried, were reactivated by the accident and by his physical dependence, he felt as if he could only survive by being strong and self-reliant, much as he had felt then and he behaved accordingly towards those whose role it was to care for him.)

and children absorb these gradually and often unconsciously. In the psychoanalytic approach, the symptoms of mental illness are seen as a by-product of the attempt to keep out of conscious awareness those impulses, urges, emotions which are seen as wicked, forbidden, or overwhelmingly painful.

This involves a great deal of psychic energy because unconscious material is, according to this theory, always striving energetically for conscious awareness where it can be processed and integrated, despite resistance, as part of the self, 'worked through', as Freud described it. When, for whatever reason, the defence mechanisms which maintain the material at an unconscious level, begin to falter, the resulting anxiety and the renewed and increasingly desperate attempts to keep the material unconscious are made manifest in symptoms of mental illness or psychological disturbance. Therefore, someone who prides themselves on being very strong and independent and believes it is weak to be distressed or need help, may struggle with enormous conflict if something major occurs in their life in which the need for help and support is vital. Someone who feels it is wrong to be angry and resentful may struggle when something really significant happens that understandably elicits such emotions.

'Aspects of ourselves which conflict with consciously held ideals may be denied, suppressed or disowned and become more or less unconscious' (Brown and Pedder 1991: 14).

Giving a form to our mental life through symbolisation, expressing our ideas and feelings to another person who listens and accepts them helps us to own those ideas and feelings, to manage them and integrate them as part of our experience

Nicholls (2003) argues that strong emotions are normal and usual for those who have had suffered injury, loss and serious illness and should not be regarded as indicative of some pathological process. Healthcare workers may feel uncomfortable and helpless when strong emotions are expressed by patients, especially if they feel they should be able to prevent or quell them and solve the problems they see as causing them. Yet we talk about needing to get things off our chests and about not bottling them up and it is those experiences that are most emotionally charged that we seem to need to verbalise. Sugarman (2006) points out that the ability to verbalise our inner world and inner processes can both prevent and alleviate symptoms and behavioural patterns that are maladaptive. Speaking about what has happened to us, having someone to bear witness to our story, its significance for us and what we feel about it, is important. Symbolising it, through words, makes it more real. This helps us to begin to accept and integrate the experience and the accompanying emotions as part of ourselves and our own history. Therefore, the expression of thoughts, impulses and emotions, and the fact that they are heard, even encouraged (although never forced) and understood by another human being, who can bear them and accept them, is, in itself, the beginning of a healing process that promotes mental health. Malan (1995 p.3) asks a crucial question:

How many patients present themselves at GP's surgeries, or psychiatric out-patient departments and are given a diagnosis of 'depression' (for which the treatment is anti-depressants) or 'anxiety' (for which the treatment is tranquillizers) when the true diagnosis is unexpressed painful feelings. . . . ?

Leader and Corfield (2007: 292) discuss the importance of being able to symbolise our experiences. They argue that 'the more we are taken up into symbolic, linguistic structures, the more the experience of the body in pain can be mediated. We can talk about it, ask for help, give a meaning to it and so on'.

The psychodynamic approach, and the psychoanalytic theories on which it is based have many critics. One criticism often levelled at it is that is not falsifiable and that its scientific basis can never be truly established. Indeed, any criticism of it can be interpreted, in a circular argument as arising from unconscious hostility. Frosh (1999: 234) pointed that it is not 'a discipline in which immaculate and uncontaminated evidence is available for rational and judicious scrutiny'.

However, the assumption that this is possible in any scientific discipline is questionable and very much depends on how one defines science. There is a growing belief that the positivistic approach, in its attempt to discover objective, impartial and unbiased evidence is not always the most valid framework for studying the complexities and contradictions of humans beings. The ways in which we experience events and situations and the meanings we attribute to them are increasingly seen as more fruitful areas of investigation (Willig 2001). A psychodynamic approach takes an interpretivist stance in which the subjectivity of psychodynamic theory and practice and also of patient and carer is acknowledged and is indeed central.

A cognitive-behavioural approach to mental health

The cognitive-behavioural approach to mental health is in many ways very different from the psychoanalytic approach yet as this perspective evolves, some of the boundaries between the two approaches appear to be blurring. It is currently a popular and recommended approach for many mental health problems (DH 2004) because of its strong evidence base. I have chosen to include it in this chapter because I believe some of its principles and techniques, explained below, can inform all healthcare professionals from all disciplines and in all clinical areas about the importance of their communication with clients in promoting mental health.

1. *The cognitive behavioural approach to mental health rests on the premise that a significant factor in the development and maintenance of mental health is the conscious meaning that we attach to events and the impact of this on our emotions and on our learned responses to situations.*

In even the most tranquil and contented life there will be difficulties and losses. The interpretation or meaning that is given to these can significantly affect mental health. The death of a much loved wife/husband/partner, for example, is one of the most profound losses that can be experienced. The surviving partner will have to make huge readjustments to his or her life, whatever the circumstances, and is likely to feel a range of intense and difficult emotions over a long period. Some people will realise that these feelings will eventually fade or become bearable and that they will, with time and support, adjust to their new circumstances. Others may believe that they will never recover and that no future happiness is possible. For the latter, depression and anxiety are much more likely. We all hold deeply ingrained beliefs about ourselves, about the world and about other people which have a major impact on our emotions and behaviour. For us all, the conscious meaning we attribute to an event, our beliefs about it and the context in which it occurs, have a major influence on the emotions it elicits (Beck 1976). See Box 7.2.

Box 7.2 Example of meaning and context affecting emotions

1. There is a loud knock on the door of your house in the remote countryside, on a dark night when you are in alone and expecting no one.

2. There is a loud knock on the door of your house in the remote countryside on a dark night when you are in alone. Someone who lives with you has recently telephoned to say that they will be home shortly and that they don't have their key with them.

Discussion points

How much anxiety do you think you would you experience in the first scenario? Rate it from 0 to 10, where 10 represents the highest level you can imagine.

How much anxiety do you think you would you experience in the second scenario? Rate it from 0 to 10, where 10 represents the highest level you can imagine.

Presumably, you will have rated the knock on the door in the first scenario as much more scary than the knock on the door in the second. The information you had about the event and the context in which it occurred directly affected your emotional reaction to it. It might also affect your behaviour in that you would probably be much more likely to answer the door in the second scenario than in the first.

2. People sometimes draw faulty conclusions about themselves, other people and the world in general. These are called cognitive distortions and they can maintain low mood and anxiety and affect behaviour and its reinforcements.

There are so many ways in which the most well-delivered information can be affected and distorted by anxious and vulnerable patients. One fear-laden word like 'cancer' for example, may raise a patient's anxieties to a level which prevents them from attending to the rest of the information. Some patients' anxieties may be temporarily reduced by 'selective listening' in which only the positive aspects of the message are heard and their expectations are unrealistic. In even the most neutral or benign of circumstances, recall of information is imperfect. When we are in pain, and anxious about our health and when serious injury or disease has challenged our view of ourselves and our future, we revert to more primitive thinking which impedes our ability to reflect on situations realistically and to solve problems.

Information giving is rightly seen as a crucial aspect of communication in healthcare. What patients are told about their illness, injury or disease will affect the meaning it has for them. Accurate information, given in a sensitive and timely manner, has many functions:

- understanding current symptoms
- understanding possible treatments
- understanding the prognosis
- understanding how much adjustment to one's lifestyle may be required
- being able to make informed decisions about different treatments and/or about the end of life and dying.

This all implies that once the patient has been given accurate well-delivered information, on a single occasion, albeit supplemented by written material, they will recall it, reliably and perfectly. We know, however, that human beings just aren't like that. Our thinking can become distorted in different ways, which is why the patient's reaction to the information given and their ongoing grasp and understanding of their situation, which can of course change, need to be repeatedly checked (Nicholls 2003). Without such information the conclusions we reach about what is happening and its implications for the future may be unrealistic and inaccurate, leading to thoughts which are not

Box 7.3 Example of distorted thinking

Freya had had a long and painful illness from which she had gradually recovered. She had tried to return to work before she was physically ready and she had to take further sick leave. She reluctantly gave up her job but missed the camaraderie of her colleagues and the self-esteem she gained through doing her work well. When she was physically well enough to look for another post, the anxiety she had developed about using the bus, her main form of transport, prevented her from travelling to employment agencies in the city centre. Her mood lowered, she became clinically depressed and she was referred to a community psychiatric nurse (CPN).

As part of a cognitive-behavioural programme, she and the CPN travelled on the bus together and explored the exact nature of her fears. She said the worst part of the journey was when they were stuck in heavy traffic. She imagined that she might have a full-blown panic attack, despite never having had one. It emerged that her anxiety-laden thinking processes led her to believe that if she did have a panic attack, she would be taken to a psychiatric hospital, treated badly and possibly never allowed to leave. The worry about a single panic attack, which had never actually occurred, led to her thinking she might be locked away, never to be released! These negative thoughts were explored and their validity gently challenged.

only unhelpful in terms of our motivation and physical recovery but which may also lead to unnecessary anxiety and depression. See Box 7.3.

This is an example of a *cognitive distortion* called *catastrophising*, an incorrect conclusion in which a catastrophic outcome is envisaged from a relatively insignificant occurrence. Another frequently occurring example of distorted thinking includes drawing conclusions on the basis of a single incident, on little evidence or even on evidence to the contrary (*arbitrary influence*) Someone who is learning to walk again following a road traffic accident, for example, may tell themselves, when they stumble or struggle, that they will never walk again despite the fact that they are making good progress.

A further example is the tendency to view events, other people or oneself in polarised terms (*dichotomous thinking*). The person learning to walk again may believe that they are either completely healthy and able bodied or totally useless and worthless.

3. Cognitive distortions can be revealed when negative automatic thoughts are identified.

I have just suggested, in the example given above, that the person learning to walk again may 'tell themself' something, for example, they may say to themselves, 'This is hopeless, I'll never walk again.' This is an example of *an automatic negative thought*. We are all thinking constantly, in a stream of consciousness, about what we are doing, about what we are going to do, about the experiences we have had. These thoughts, which often pass through our minds so quickly that we may hardly be aware of them, can have a significant influence on our mood. Greenberger and Padesky (1995) point out that such thoughts can also be in the form of mental images, so that the person struggling to walk again may think 'this is hopeless, I'll never walk again' but they may also have an image of themselves in a highly dependent state in a wheelchair, being stared at and pitied. Such negative thoughts and images can present themselves, rapidly and unbidden, particularly when we are in a negative frame of mind, which is more likely when we are ill or injured. The lowered mood that follows will make it harder for patients to motivate themselves for their rehabilitation and harder to test out the validity of their mood-lowering, automatic thoughts through their actions. See Box 7.4.

A technique that can be used to encourage patients to consider their answers to these kind of questions is *Socratic questioning*, so named because it is based on the teaching methods of the early Greek philosopher Socrates. Carey and Mullan (2004) point out that there are many discrepancies in the literature about the purpose and

---

Box 7.4 Check point

The next time you have a strong emotional reaction to an event or interaction with someone, it can be useful to consider what automatic thoughts preceded or accompanied it. Ask yourself the following questions:

- What was going through my mind before I started to feel this way?
- What does this say about me if it is true?
- What does this mean about me, my life, my future?
- What am I afraid might happen?
- What is the worst thing that could happen if it is true?
- What does this mean about how other people think about me?
- What does this mean about the other person or people in general?
- What images or memories do I have in this situation?

(Adapted from Greenberger and Padesky 1995).

technique of Socratic questioning, despite its being a well-established psychotherapeutic procedure. I am using the term here to describe a form of questioning which encourages reflection on the possibly faulty assumptions that are being made. The person whose negative automatic thoughts are being considered is not directly told that their thoughts and assumptions may be faulty or inaccurate (as in 'of course you will walk again, you must think positively, look how well you are doing!) but rather, the validity of their thoughts, assumptions and conclusions is explored through focused questioning. Examples of the questions that may be asked include: How sure are you of that? How likely is that ? What is the evidence to support that thought? What evidence to the contrary is there? What alternative explanations are there? What would I say to a good friend who was coming to this conclusion? What has helped in the past?

Such probing questions, asked gently, at an appropriate time and pace, help the person to discover and process for themselves, possible alternative ways of thinking about their situation. This is likely to be far more meaningful than simply being told what to think, in a way which closes down communication.

I am not suggesting, however, that all patients' negative thoughts are distorted and should be challenged. They may have realistic perceptions of what their illness or injury means for them, for their future and their relationships. Having someone to talk to about this can be an important part of adjusting to their changed circumstances, of assessing what help is needed and of making the most of what is possible.

One of the reasons for the current popularity of the cognitive behavioural approach to mental health is the evidence base for its efficacy (the positive effects it has in clinical trials). As Holmes (2002) explains, psychoanalysis, from which the psychodynamic approach derives, has been slow to acknowledge the necessity of demonstrating its credibility and worth.

However, the cognitive behavioural approach can be criticised for its assumption that human beings are, at heart, logical and rational and that low mood and anxiety will inevitably be alleviated by more accurate and balanced thinking. Although this is often the case, humans also have complex internal dynamics, irrational fantasies, motives and impulses which are not necessarily amenable to logical challenge. Holmes (2002) questions the evidence for the use of cognitive behaviour therapy in actual clinical practice despite its seeming efficacy in clinical trials. What does emerge consistently from investigation into the different approaches to psychotherapy is that the nature of the relationship between client and therapist is hugely important and the best predictor of outcome (Horvarth and Symonds 1991). This could be seen as implying that the specific 'techniques' of each approach are of minor importance, conversely, perhaps, it suggests that sound technique involves providing the kind of relationship that is optimum for that person at that time. For patients struggling with pain, disability and disease, the fact that a healthcare professional is sufficiently caring and motivated to attempt an exploration of how they think and feel about their situation and then to listen, understand and accept their thoughts and feelings, however difficult to hear these may be, can be therapeutic in itself.

Both the psychodynamic and the cognitive behavioural approaches to mental health are collaborative, 'person-centred' approaches in as much that both recognise, albeit at different levels, that 'what matters is the way an event is registered in the particular and highly specific history of a unique person' (Leader and Corfield 2007: 52). Both approaches include reasons for and ways of communicating which can be integrated into the care of psychologically vulnerable clients by any healthcare professional with a positive attitude to promoting mental health. See Box 7.5.

Box 7.5 Vignette of a lost opportunity for promoting mental health

Carol, a 54 year old woman, had had a mastectomy 4 months ago. She had recovered well from the surgery, and the consultant oncologist who had later seen her in out-patients had been very patient and explained clearly the results of all the tests and their implications. She had even given Carol a little hug after she had told her that all the lymph glands were clear and there was no evidence of any spread of the cancer. 'You are very lucky' she said.

When Carol went to the hospital for her first cycle of chemotherapy, she talked to other women who had had mastectomies. Some had malignant cells in their lymph glands, some had larger tumours removed. 'I am very lucky,' she thought.

At first, the chemotherapy just made her feel tired. She persevered with the second and third cycle of chemotherapy, when she lost her hair and felt sick but during the fourth cycle she was admitted to hospital with an infection. She felt weak, shivery and exhausted and when her husband, who had been ill himself, and her son Ben came to visit, they were very concerned and loving. Ben had recently moved to London to a new job. She tried to put on a brave face so as not to upset them.

(Continued overleaf)

She thought about her friend from work, Janet, who had died last year from pancreatic cancer. She used to really enjoy talking to Janet, she could always say anything to her. Janet had been brave and cheerful to the end.

Later, after all the visitors on the ward had gone, Carol sat in the chair by her bed. Her newspaper had slipped to the floor and she leaned forward, but then felt too exhausted to bend right down to pick it up. She caught a glimpse down her nightdress, of the scar where her breast had been. She tried, unsuccessfully, to blink back the tears. At almost the same moment, the night sister, recently arrived on duty, came into her room and said 'Hello, how are you feeling this evening?' and then picked up the newspaper for her. She noticed Carol's tears and she stopped at the door. 'Oh dear,' she said, 'are you feeling a bit down? You'll feel better once we have got to grips with this infection and you can go home. Let us know if you need anything, won't you?' Carol swallowed her tears, nodded, and even managed a wan smile. The sister closed the door behind her.

Discussion points

1. What losses has Carol recently experienced?
2. What emotions might you expect her to have as a result?
3. What thoughts might be going through her mind?
4. What messages, perhaps unintentionally, were the consultant oncologist and the ward sister giving Carol about those emotions and thoughts?
5. Why might they be giving her this message?
6. How might the ward sister have reacted in order to better promote Carol's mental health?

Communication skills training

I hope that I have given a convincing explanation of how good communication in healthcare settings contributes to patients' mental health. I also hope that gaining some increased understanding will motivate healthcare professionals to take the learning and teaching of communications skills very seriously. These have long been included and emphasised in both the pre- and post-registration training and education of healthcare professionals. Despite this, Chant et al. (2002), in their literature review of communication skills training in nurse education, found that there were few research studies evaluating such training and that many of these were methodologically flawed. Reynolds et al. (1999) challenge the underpinning premise of communication skills training, which is that students can transfer their learning to clinical practice with real patients. Communication skills training is usually evaluated on the basis of subjective reports of students, and its observable impact on skills in real-life clinical situations is more difficult to assess.

Freshwater and Stickley (2004) suggest that communication skills taught as a discrete activity, much like giving an injection, is unsatisfactory because it separates communication from genuine caring and empathy and presents it as yet another set of technical skills, divorced from real emotional connection with the patient. However, Skelton (2005: 40), discussing communications skills training in medical education, argues that time is being wasted debating such questions and that 'common sense and everyday experience tells us that skills are indeed improved by training and practice'. He claims that a more important question is about how such skills are deployed, about whether a focus on skills training leads to desirable attitudes or whether teaching appropriate attitudes generates the necessary skills.

This initially seems to be a false dichotomy, in that healthcare professionals need to develop both desirable attitudes and sound communication skills, but it does illuminate an important point. Most of us can learn certain verbal and non-verbal behaviours, such as active listening, using different types of questions, clarifying, making empathic statements, reflecting and so on. However, skilled performance of this repertoire of behaviours (which involves using them with the right person, in the right context, in the right way and at the right time) requires a positive attitude to engaging with patients in this way.

Social psychologists conceptualise attitudes as being comprised of cognitions, emotions and behaviour (Stratton and Hayes 1993). The healthcare professional must therefore believe that employing these skilled behaviours will make a difference (*the cognitive dimension*), feel reasonably positive and confident about doing so, (*the emotional dimension*), before they will actually attempt to use the skills in clinical practice (*the behavioural dimension*).

The consequences of our communication with patients, be it excellent, average or poor, are often not immediately observable. The impact may be subtle and gradual, as with the messages parents give their children. This lack of immediate and easily discernible feedback makes it more difficult for us to identify good and poor communication in the clinical arena and to recognise its influence.

Simulated patients

One way in which this can be addressed is by practising with simulated patients. Simulated patients, actors taking on the role of patients, are encouraged to reflect on and give prompt and specific feedback about the nuances of the communication received and how it affects them (Rees et al. 2004). This takes place in a safe environment in which skills can be rehearsed and mistakes made, without adverse consequences for real patients.

Rollnick et al. (2002) have argued for the effectiveness of what they called 'context-bound communication' with experienced medical practitioners, in their place of work. The emphasis was on improving one's handling of everyday clinical situations identified as difficult by practitioners (with the use of paid actors as simulated patients), rather than on communication skills per se. The notion that the practitioners were in some way deficient in their performance of communication skills was rejected, in favour of a need to improve skills already in place but severely tested by specific situations. The authors claimed success for this approach partly because it proved acceptable to the clinicians, a highly desirable state of affairs.

There is, however, a disadvantage to focusing communications skills training only on situations which the practitioner has identified as difficult. Awareness should also be raised of the critical aspects of communication in interactions which may not be obviously and immediately challenging, yet which have a significant impact on the patient. When an emotional reaction in a patient is ignored, dismissed or blocked, what may be communicated is that the expression of that emotion is inappropriate or unacceptable in the present context, perhaps because it is perceived as unmanageable or unimportant, weak, embarrassing or shameful. The impact of this crucial message may not be instantly discernible, but can be very powerful nevertheless.

The need to communicate

The human tendency to tell others about what has happened to us, the wish for others to bear witness to our experience, may be reflected in the current appetite for blogs, Youtube videos and camera phones. McCleod (2007: 146) states that 'when a person experiences a stressful or difficult situation in their life, there seems to be a natural tendency to want to tell the story of these events to at least one other person'. He cites the work of Pennebaker (1997) who found in a series of studies that groups of volunteers, who disclosed, albeit briefly, their experience of stressful events for the purpose of the study, and who were measured at various points during the studies, scored more highly on a range of measures related to health and happiness than the control groups who had not engaged in any disclosure for the study.

McCleod suggests that when people are inhibited, for whatever reason, in their need to tell others about their experiences, they have higher levels of autonomic arousal which can become stressful and interfere with information processing and with assimilation of those experiences.

As health professionals we can learn to bear witness to the stories of our patients, to really listen, to show some understanding and acceptance of how their illness or injury has affected them, what it means to them and how they are coping with it. If we also appreciate how and why this is crucial and we apply our learning in practice, we can then claim to have truly engaged in mental health promotion.

- The perceptions of what constitutes mental health and mental illness are in part dependent on the culture and values of the society we live in.
- Healthcare professionals both create and reflect a specific culture and values, which they communicate very subtly to their patients at a period in their lives when they may be particularly vulnerable to the development of mental health problems.
- The psychodynamic approach to mental health emphasises the importance of unconscious processes and the need for feelings and impulses to be consciously acknowledged, spoken of, understood and accepted by other human beings.
- The cognitive-behavioural approach focuses on how responses are learnt and the impact of thoughts on emotions and behaviour. It considers the ways in which information can be processed and sometimes distorted, leading to inaccurate conclusions affecting adjustment and recovery which the healthcare professional can sensitively explore and challenge.
- Healthcare practitioners' communication with their clients can be improved with skills training but frameworks for understanding the value of skilled communication in promoting mental health are needed to raise the motivation and confidence of practitioners to put the skills into practice.

References

Anderson S.M. and Miranda R. (2000) Transference. How past relationships emerge in the present. *The Psychologist* 13(12): 608–9.

Beck A.T. (1976) *Cognitive Therapy and the Emotional Disorders.* New York: International Universities Press.

Bee P., Richards D., Loftus S., Baker J., Bailey L., Lovell K., Woods P. and Cox D. (2006) Mapping nursing activity in acute inpatient mental health-care settings. *Journal of Mental Health* 15(2): 217–26.

Brown D. and Pedder J. (1991) *Introduction to Psychotherapy.* London: Routledge.

Carey T.A. and Mullan R.J. (2004) What is Socratic Questioning? *Psychotherapy Research, Practice, Training* 41(3): 217–26.

Chant S., Jenkinson T., Randle J., Russell G. and Webb C. (2002) Communications skills training in healthcare: a review of the literature. *Nurse Education Today* 22: 189–202.

Davis H. and Fallowfield L. (1991) *Counselling and Communication in Healthcare.* Chichester: Wiley.

Department of Health (DH) (2004) *Organising and Delivering Psychological Therapies.* London: HMSO.

Ellenberger H.F. (1970) *The Discovery of the Unconscious: the history and evolution of dynamic psychiatry.* New York: Basic Books.

Freshwater D. (2006) *Mental Health and Illness: Questions and Answers for Counsellors and Therapists.* Chichester: Whurr.

Freshwater D. and Stickley T. (2004) The heart of the art: emotional intelligence in nurse education. *Nursing Inquiry* 11(2): 91–8.

Freud S. (1923) The Ego and the Id. In J. Strachey (ed. and trans.) *The Standard Edition of the complete psychological works of Sigmund Freud* Standard Edition, Vol 19. London: Hogarth, pp. 1–60.

Freud S. (1925) An Autobiographical Study. In Strachey (ed. and trans.) *The Standard Edition of the Complete Psychological Works of Sigmund Freud,* Standard Edition, Vol 20. London: Hogarth, pp. 1–74.

Freud S. (1958) The dynamics of transference. In Strachey (ed. and trans.) *The Standard Edition of the Complete Psychological Works of Sigmund Freud,* Vol 12. London: Hogarth, pp. 97–108.

Frosh S. (1999) *The Politics of Psychoanalysis: an introduction to Freudian and post-Freudian theory.* Basingstoke: Macmillan.

Greenberger D. and Padesky C.A. (1995) *Mind Over Mood.* New York: Guilford Press.

Holmes J. (2002) All you need is cognitive-behaviour therapy? *British Medical Journal* 324: 288–94.

Horvath A. and Symonds D. (1991) Relationship between working alliance and outcome in psychotherapy: a meta-analysis. *Journal of Counselling Psychology* 38: 139–49.

Leader D. and Corfield D. (2007) *Why do People get Ill?* London: Hamish Hamilton.

London School of Economics (LSE) (2006) *The Depression Report. A New Deal for Depression and Anxiety Disorders.* London: Centre for Economic Performance's Mental Health Policy Group.

Malan D.H. (1995) *Individual Psychotherapy and the Science of Psychodynamics.* Oxford: Butterworth-Heinemann.

McCleod J. (2007) *Counselling Skill.* Maidenhead: Open University Press.

Nicholls K. (2003) *Psychological Care for Ill and Injured People – A Clinical Guide.* Maidenhead: Open University Press.

Nursing and Midwifery Council (NMC) (2002) *Practitioner–client Relationships and the Prevention of Abuse.* London: NMC.

Pennebaker J.W. (1997) *Opening Up: The Healing Power of Expressing Emotions.* New York: Guildford Press.

Power M. (2000) Freud and the unconscious. *The Psychologist* 13(12): 612–14.

Rees C., Sheard C. and McPherson A. (2004) Medical students' views and experiences of methods of teaching and learning communication skills. *Patient Education and Counseling* 54: 119–21.

Reynolds W.J., Scott B. and Jessima W. (1999) Empathy has not been measured in clients' terms or effectively taught: a review of the literature. *Journal of Advanced Nursing* 30(5): 1177–85.

Rinomhota S. and Marshall P. (2000) *Biological Aspects of Mental Health Nursing.* London: Churchill Livingstone.

Rollnick S., Kinnersley P. and Butler C. (2002) Context-bound communication skills training: development of a new method. *Medical Education* 36: 377–83.

Skelton J.R. (2005) Everything you were afraid to ask about communication skills. *British Journal of General Practice* 55: 40–6.

Stratton P. and Hayes N. (1993) *A Student's Dictionary of Psychology.* London: Edward Arnold.

Sugarman A. (2006) Mentalization, insightfulness, and therapeutic action. The importance of mental organization. *International Journal of Psychoanalysis* 87: 965–87.

Whittington D. and McLaughlin C. (2000) Finding time for patients: an exploration of nurses' time allocation in an acute psychiatric setting. *Journal of Psychiatric and Mental Health Nursing* 7: 259–68.

Willig C. (2001) *Qualitative Research in Psychology.* Buckingham: Open University Press.

World Health Organization (WHO) (2001) *Strengthening Mental Health Promotion* (fact sheet no. 20). Geneva: World Health Organization.

World Health Organization (WHO) (2005) *Promoting Mental Health.* Geneva: World Health Organization.

Chapter 8

The impact of childhood chronic illness and disability on family life

Jenny Waite-Jones

Introduction

Whilst a general discussion of chronic illness and related interventions was offered in Chapter 3, specific consideration is given within this chapter to how childhood chronic illness and disability impacts on family relationships. The experiences of different family members over the family life-cycle are explored and, as families are embedded in a network of social relationships, including extended family, friends and neighbours, the extent to which these can prove supportive is also discussed. In addition, current initiatives, which recognise the need to see ill and disabled child patients within their family, and community context, are also considered.

Although there is a need within current healthcare provision generally to acknowledge the role of a patient's family, and community experiences, in their health status, this is particularly important when considering child health and well-being, as the extent to which patient and professional partnerships can be formed is dependent upon the child's age and abilities. Attempts by professionals to form such partnerships are much more likely to be aimed at parents, and, thus, have a more indirect effect on the child than those possible with adult patients. Children are particularly dependent upon their parents and other family members, and such relationships will heavily influence their experiences of illness and disability. It is, thus, important to consider influences of childhood illness and disability on family life, and how individuals respond to such experiences.

Childhood chronic illness and disability and family life

It is important to see children with chronic conditions within their family context as such relationships influence how individuals understand and structure their lives, and gain a sense of 'who they are' (Hockney and James 2003). Whilst aware that current family structures vary, it is only possible within one chapter to consider 'the family' in terms defined by Gittins (1993) as, 'kinship' ties between related individuals through birth and mating, usually involving co-residency with divisions based on power through gendered and age related roles. However, family function, irrespective of the actual structure, helps to provide physical and emotional security, whilst promoting development of individual identity. Successful family function includes flexible adaptation to developmental demands and coping with events threatening the ability of the family to provide for its members (Bradford 1997).

Bronfenbrenner's (1979: 2005) bio-ecological approach, outlined in Chapter 3, is particularly useful in explaining how relationships within the child's micro-system, including family, extended family, peers, school and healthcare professionals, as well as interactions between these different components (meso-system), impact upon health and well-being. Family experiences dominate a child's micro-system, as the family, itself a system balancing the needs of individual members, includes strong emotional ties with the distress of one member affecting others (Dallos and Draper 2006). For example, Anthony et al. (2003) found a relationship between parents' perceptions of vulnerability in their ill child and levels of anxiety expressed by children with arthritis. Also, Schanberg et al. (2001) found that the way parents express pain is related to pain perception and behaviour in children with chronic rheumatic disease.

How children perceive and respond to having a chronic illness and/or disability can influence their psychological and physical well-being. Bradford (1997) suggests that even young children develop scripts concerning illness and treatment behaviour, and that how they think and feel about their situation impacts on their behaviour. An understanding of the relationship between stress and chronic conditions discussed in Chapter 3 is equally pertinent here. For example, daily difficulties have been identified as stressful for children with juvenile arthritis (von Weiss et al. 2002).

Stress on family members

The whole family may experience stress in different ways. Gerhardt et al. (2003) point out that juvenile idiopathic arthritis (JIA) has the potential to disrupt family functioning as parents face uncertainty, lack of control, and pressures from the daily difficulties of caring for an ill child. Also, Mescon and Honig (1995) found parental fatigue resulting from caring for children with various conditions, including diabetes and cancer, with fathers suffering depression, ulcers, headaches and obesity, and mothers prone to depression and other psychological illnesses. Many parents feel helpless, powerless and isolated. Mothers have less opportunity to work outside the home, whilst fathers work longer hours to support their family. The loss of leisure time within the family may impact upon the siblings, as parents are preoccupied with their ill child (Britton 2001; Waite-Jones and Madill 2008a).

Whilst families of children with chronic illness and disabilities face similar experiences, the nature of the condition can also create specific concerns. For example, the extreme variability, unpredictability, occasional invisibility of symptoms and lack of understanding of JIA creates particularly stressful circumstances including a loss of credibility through not being believed (Britton 2001). Also, Edwards and Davis (1997) suggest that rare conditions bring additional stresses through lack of understanding and relevant support.

Bradford (1997) defines family adjustment as the ability to engage in age appropriate tasks, lack of sick role behaviour, and accepting limitations of the condition positively. However, such factors are influenced by wider issues involving how individuals perceive they are seen, and judged, by others including family, healthcare professionals and those within their wider social network (Barlow et al. 1998), as well as finance, emotional support, communication and levels of healthcare available (Mescon and Honig 1995). All of these factors may, also, be experienced differently across the family life-cycle (Bennett et al. 1996).

Moreover, family members may perceive and react differently to the same family event. Accounts of children's experiences of chronic conditions offered by parents have differed from those of their child (Le-Bovidge et al. 2003), and parents often do not notice adverse reactions of siblings. Rather than treat family members' experiences as homogenous, it is necessary to consider how childhood chronic illness and disability affects different family members. As their interpretation of family events will be coloured by expectations based on experiences outside the home (Dunn 2000) reflecting broader social perceptions, it is useful to consider how chronic illness and disability affects the ill child, siblings and parents.

Children's experiences of chronic illness and disability

Chronic illness and disability can affect all aspects of a child's life. For example, Dixon-Wood (2007) explains how experiencing cancer, now considered a childhood chronic illness due to the high survival rate, has the potential to influence psychological, social and economic aspects of a child's later life. Beattie and Lewis-Jones (2006) also report children with chronic skin conditions as experiencing similar psychosocial problems as those with conditions such as cerebral palsy, renal failure and cystic fibrosis. Having a chronic condition can mean experiencing pain, disability and increased interactions with adults, particularly health professionals, which may enhance emotional maturity yet create greater dependency on others (Guell 2007). Also, mood swings can result from certain kinds of medication and produce negative responses from others (Britton and Moore 2002). How children manage the physical and psychosocial effects of chronic illness/disability is influenced by the visibility of their condition, their age and particular stage of development.

Children experiencing pain from an early age may see this as 'normal', and express their pain differently to adults, often denying pain when this is obviously the case. Young children in pain may be seen as 'miserable' moody, picky with food and un-manageable, yet undergo a remarkable personality change once their pain is treated (Britton and Moore 2002).

Chronic conditions can also bring restricted mobility, irritability, aggression, hope and despair (Sallfors et al. 2002), and as children mature those with visibly worse conditions may become withdrawn due to experiencing difficult social relationships (Reiter-Purtill et al. 2003). Teachers report fewer behavioural problems from children with severe conditions, but may well make special allowances denied to those with less obvious signs of illness/disability. For example, teachers rated children with obvious signs of juvenile arthritis as less aggressive and disruptive than those whose condition was less obvious, who they described as moody and picky (Sturge et al. 1997). However, lenient treatment offered by teachers and other adults to those with obvious disability is often resented as it can make them feel even more different to their peers (Waite-Jones 2005).

Appearance and well-being

Changes to a child's physical appearance may be due to side effects of their medication as well as the condition itself. For example, Laxer

(1999) found adverse psychological effects of steroids due to the short stature, weight gain and cushingoid features these can create. Price (1993) describes the relationship between self-esteem and body image, with differences and similarities measured against others and a 'goodness of fit' model applied which becomes increasingly sophisticated through childhood and adolescence. Children and adolescents with the most visible physical differences are at risk of developing a low self-esteem due to their perceived poor self-image (Dahlquist 2003) and likely to exhibit depressive symptoms (Wallander and Varni 1998). (See Chapter 5 for more detail on self-image and self-esteem).

Children least visibly affected by their condition may face different, but equally difficult social barriers (Barlow et al. 1998). Less visible symptoms can mean being teased for poor physical performance and receiving mixed messages from parents, doctors and others as to what is expected of them (MacLeod 1995). Whilst children with mild symptoms look similar to their peers, those with more obvious signs of chronic illness/disability have to accept their condition on an everyday level and develop appropriate coping mechanisms (White 1996). Children with the less visible symptoms possibly strive to pass as healthy but experience constant reminders that this is not the case. Experiencing a chronic condition can be seen as a continuum, with those displaying visible signs more believed but feeling physically different, whilst those with less physical signs may not so look different but face greater disbelief. Thus, experiences at both ends of the spectrum mean feeling different, but in different ways.

Social acceptance

Being more mature for their years, due to experiencing a medical condition involving many interactions with adults, yet, at times, physically and socially more dependent than their peers, can make 'same age' social relationships difficult for older children and adolescents with chronic conditions. For example, those suffering a brain tumour (Upton and Eiser 2006) and fibromyalgia syndrome (Kashikar-Zuck et al. 2007) reported experiencing problematic peer relationships.

Children with chronic conditions may feel inadequate, suffer emotional problems and display poor social skills resulting in bullying from their peers (Krulik and Florian 1995). For example, social rejection and problematic behaviour have been linked to levels of depression in those with juvenile rheumatic diseases, even when controlling for levels of pain (Sandstrom and Schonberg 2004). Such children also may see their physical difference as a stigma which may be contagious for those who associate with them (Waite-Jones 2005).

Social acceptance is so important that older children and adolescents work hard to conceal their condition and if possible live a life similar to their peers (Huygen et al. 2000). However, concealing symptoms of the condition can perpetuate the lack of understanding, which contributes negative peer response. An optimal amount of openness and concealment is required, as enough of the former is necessary to let others know that special consideration is in order, but too much can be construed as sympathy seeking (Waite-Jones 2005).

Challenges created by the education system

Inflexibility within the compulsory education system can increase the pain and fatigue experienced by children with chronic conditions. Problems become more pronounced for those transferring to secondary education, which coincides with adolescence, a stage already requiring great psychological and physiological adjustment. The size and related organisation of secondary schools mean more rigid rules and regulations as well as exposure of difference to a greater number of peers. Increased experiences of bullying in secondary schools suggest that the hierarchical nature of such institutions provides a context whereby the response to 'difference' can be bullying. However, the structure of college and university life helps in overcoming past difficult experiences and improving self-esteem (Schafer et al. 2004). Vulnerability to feeling 'different' reduces over time through cessation of compulsory education and greater self-understanding and maturity of peers when those with chronic conditions approach adulthood (Waite-Jones 2005).

Achieving independence

Achieving the independence normally expected during adolescence can be difficult for those with a chronic condition. Even though they have the cognitive capacity to comply with medical regimes, compliance may be influenced negatively by the desire to behave like healthy peers (McDonagh et al. 2000). Young people also need to maintain good family relationships to help them manage their condition. For example, Straughair (1992) describes how one girl was unable to remove her socks for three days after a family argument. However, they may be placed in a paradoxical position, in that they may require family assistance, as well as support from other agencies, to become independent of their family (Huygen et al. 2000).

Those with chronic conditions, such as JIA, may be disadvantaged during adulthood in terms of education and employment (Peterson et al. 1997; Woo and Wedderburn 1998). However, such a future may not always be so bleak as Arkela-Kautianen et al. (2005) found young adults with JIA comparable with health peers in terms of unemployment, education and spousal relationships.

Adjustment to childhood chronic conditions is facilitated by social support in the form of family and peers (von Weiss et al. 2002), as well as the adoption of a measured openness in explaining to others about the condition.

Siblings' experiences

When a child has a chronic illness/disability it is important to understand their siblings' experiences too, given the children's potential to share the longest of all relationships which is integrated within a family network and impacts upon adjustment and self-identity (Dunn 2000). For example, well siblings are often distressed on their ill sibling's behalf. Batte et al. (2006) and Harding (1996) found that the emotional response of siblings of children with cancer could be as strong as that of their ill brother or sister as that they often felt neglected and unhappy.

Adverse effects on siblings are generally reported more by parents than siblings themselves. For example, Sharpe and Rossiter (2002) found that parents of children with a number of conditions, including cancer, diabetes, cystic fibrosis and hearing problems, reported adverse effects on siblings. These different accounts were thought to be due to parents being overprotective and siblings' lack of awareness of the difficulties they were experiencing. However, siblings may have been reluctant to admit negative experiences, so as to appear as if they were coping well, and protect their family (Silver and Frohlinger-Graham 2000; Ratcliffe 2001).

Siblings may actually be much more aware than parents of difficult social relationships experienced by the ill brother or sister, particularly if they are near in age and attend the same school (Britton and Moore 2002; Waite-Jones and Madill 2008a). However, they can also feel confused, angry, frustrated, isolated, and ambivalent about their disabled brother or sister due to lack of information from parents (Houtzager 2004; Batte et al. 2006). Britton and Moore (2002) note that parents of children with juvenile idiopathic arthritis often have little time to keep siblings informed of the ill child's progress, and Ratcliffe (2001) found that siblings of children with a variety of conditions, including asthma, Down's Syndrome autism and deafness, do not ask for information from parents for fear of upsetting them.

Emotional challenges

Differential treatment from parents when disparities are unavoidable can mean that ambivalence within normal sibling relationships becomes amplified, and siblings feel worried, confused, angry, frustrated, isolated and uncertain that their own selfish desires have come true (Ratcliffe 2001). Siblings also may fear their own susceptibility to their brother or sister's condition (Britton and Moore 2002; Batte et al. 2006; Waite-Jones and Madill 2008a). They have to cope with competing emotional demands, modifying their behaviour in response to the obvious distress of their sibling, whilst requiring that their own needs be met. Ratcliffe (2001) found that siblings of children with chronic conditions often feel resentful, yet act as carers to become noticed and loved.

Childhood disability can create role reversal with younger children caring for their older brother or sister. It can also create a power imbalance within sibling relationships as well children can be placed in the paradoxical position of having considerable power over their ill sibling while, at the same time, used as a scapegoat for their pain and frustration. (Sloper 2000; Ratcliffe 2001; Waite-Jones and Madill 2008a).

Well siblings may also share some of the adverse social experiences of their ill brother or sister, particularly if they are younger and the age gap between siblings is small (Waite-Jones and Madill 2008a). Also, the vicarious 'medical career' they too may have to adopt and stressful, emotional experiences created through having an ill sibling can make relationships with peers difficult and impact negatively on the self-esteem of well siblings. Such experiences are felt acutely during adolescence and between same sex siblings (Miller 1996; Waite-Jones and Madill 2008a).

Support from siblings

However, healthy siblings can be a valuable source of support and the intimacy of relationships between siblings can increase within families facing the stressful experience of a child's chronic illness (Dunn 2000; Waite-Jones and Madill 2008a) and siblings have been seen as more considerate and understanding of others due to having a brother or sister with JIA (Britton and Moore 2002; Waite-Jones and Madill 2008a). Healthy siblings may even receive some, if few, compensations for having an ill brother or sister as parents and other family members attempted to redress imbalances in attention, and some siblings report having closer family relationships due to such illness (Sloper 2000; Britton and Moore 2002; Waite-Jones and Madill 2008a).

Nevertheless, as with other family members, siblings' experiences have to be seen as embedded within wider family interactions. Siblings' adaptation has been associated with a cohesive, expressive family environment and a positive relationship between the mother and the ill child (Billings et al. 1987). Moreover, relationships between siblings and other family members are influenced by the wider social context in which the family is placed, and socioeconomic forces are also influential (Williams et al. 2003).

Miller (1996) suggests that siblings' experiences be seen as a continuum moving from positive to negative at different times during the development of the sibling and their ill brother or sister. However, siblings' acceptance of their family situation, and ability to create and maintain a sense of self-identity independent of their family role, develops over time with increased maturity of both the sibling and brother or sister with a chronic condition (Waite-Jones and Madill 2008a).

Mothers' experiences

To appreciate a mother's experience of caring for a child with a chronic condition it is important to consider the cultural context in which she is placed, as role expectations in relation to motherhood are culturally and historically determined (Cunningham-Burley et al. 2006). Bronfenbrenner's (1979; 2005) bio-ecological approach, outlined in Chapter 3, is again useful here, as how motherhood is valued and perceived at a macro-level underpins policies and practices within the other systems which form the basis from which a mother judges her own competence, and is also judged by others.

A mother's situation is influenced by her particular family structure within the micro-system and expectations and support available within wider social systems. Currently, mothers in Britain can face tensions between their role of 'mother as carer' and 'mother as earner', which are entwined but also have distinct, and potentially conflicting, boundaries. Mothers may have to work hard to store up goodwill and a good reputation at work in preparation for any time they may have take off work if their child is ill (Cunningham-Burley et al. 2006).

Tension and vulnerability

Mothers of children with a chronic condition face heavy legal and moral responsibilities, including serious decisions, such as whether their child should receive surgery and/or toxic medication. Moreover, mothers may suffer anxiety and depression (Barlow et al. 2002) as balancing positive long-term effects of invasive treatments against the distressing, painful experiences these create for their child in the short term is challenging and can reduce their self-efficacy and confidence (Lustig et al. 1996). Also, Manuel (2001) found maternal well-being to be adversely influenced by the daily difficulties involved in the care of a chronically ill/disabled child. However, the mothers' level of education also influences their ability to deal successfully with such difficulties.

Further tensions are created for mothers as they have to help their child achieve autonomy and avoid dependency, yet still offer appropriate care (Williams 2002). This can prove slightly easier in relation to daughters, who are more likely to embrace independence and responsibility for self-care, but be harder for mothers of sons, who have to adopt a more hidden, vigilant role and risk being accused of 'nagging' (Williams 2002).

Mothers worry about their ill/disabled child, feel guilty they cannot do more to improve their condition and develop a degree of hyper-vigilance within their care so as to minimise their child's distress. A special bond can develop between mother and child, often with a shared 'code' existing between them to facilitate meeting the child's needs and resulting in a mother's ability to read her child's 'signals' (Sallfors and Hallberg 2003; Waite-Jones 2005). Indeed, mothers often use 'we' when referring to their child's experiences (Barlow et al. 1998; Waite-Jones 2005). Whilst this may reflect over-identification between mothers and their children, it can also be a realistic interpretation, in that mothers do share most of their child's adverse experiences.

However, professionals may misinterpret maternal hyper-vigilance, and Sallfors and Hallberg (2003) report that mothers exposed to such accusations feel angry, helpless, powerless and aware of the importance of their own role in making decisions about their child's care. Indeed, mothers' fear of being perceived by health professionals as overprotective is not unfounded as, for example, Power et al. (2003) suggest that children with severe juvenile arthritis are more at risk of having over-controlling, overprotective and intrusive mothers. However, that this study was based on a memory task which mothers were told would improve children's treatment compliance, meant that mothers of severely ill children would work hard in any way possible to ensure that their child could do well. The 'dominating mothers' assumed by Power et al. (2003) could rather be seen as the mothers' desperate attempts to find ways of encouraging their child's future adherence to treatments vital for their well-being, and, thus, trying to prepare them for future independence when responsible for their own treatment.

Conflicting demands and role constraints

Daniel et al. (2005) found mothers of ill children to be 'vigilant information processors', gathering information carefully over several years and, when some children were considered eligible for surgery to gain extra height, mothers worked hard to keep their child as fully informed as possible. Britton and Moore (2002) suggest that mothers of children with juvenile arthritis think rationally about their child's future, seeing themselves as sharing similar goals to professionals in working towards the long-term good of their child, and Sallfors and Hallberg (2003) report that mothers seek information and develop their own solutions as well as advise healthcare professionals.

That mothers are concerned that they may be over-protective suggests that they are not merely responding to the effects of their child's illness/disability, but rather actively appraising their own ability to succeed within motherhood and do what they perceive as the best for their child's long-term future. Such concerns can be understood in terms of a readiness to perceive mothers as irrational and over-emotional, as the work of Burman (1995) suggests that the linguistic slip, within British culture, from 'mothering' to 'smothering' does not seem to have a parallel in relation to 'fathering'. Mothers of children with chronic conditions seem particularly vulnerable to such labelling given the tensions they face whilst having to physically care for a child who is developing towards adolescence (Britton 2001; Sallfors and Hallberg 2003; Waite-Jones 2005).

Mothers also struggle to ensure equality of care is given the ill/disabled child and their siblings, and judge themselves as 'less than a good mother' (Britton and Moore 2002; Waite-Jones 2005). Mothers face conflict due to having reduced time and energy available for their personal and professional roles, which often means feeling less than a 'good partner' and sacrificing their own career aspirations. The ambivalence within motherhood generally identified by Baraitser and Noak, (2007) may become amplified, as mothers' needs become secondary to those of their child.

Mothers are placed in the paradoxical position of trying to encourage independence yet provide age-inappropriate care for their ill child which can be exacerbated by professionals who expect them to be the main decision maker regarding their child's care yet are critical if they respond too vigilantly. However, over time mothers' expectations of 'normal' family life changes due to the assimilation of their ill child's needs into family routines (Sallfors and Hallberg 2003; Waite-Jones 2005).

Mothers' well-being

Nevertheless, the well-being of mothers needs to be considered as they often feel isolated when providing long-term care (Tong 2001). A further paradox exists in that due to improved healthcare policies and practices children with chronic conditions can now be supported to live at home. However, in providing constant care their mothers may become isolated from the community in which they live (Yantzi et al. 2006). The family structure and cultural context can exacerbate such negative experiences for mothers. For example, mothers of chronically ill/disabled children within some ethnic groups feel isolated due to values and beliefs of their community as well as institutional barriers (Bywater et al. 2003).

The position of such mothers needs to be seen as a dynamic process, which, to some extent, is independent of the individuals involved. The position in which mothers are placed, in terms of societal expectations of the role of motherhood, is challenged by the uncertainty created by having a chronically ill/disabled child. Understanding and supporting mothers also helps the ill child. Appreciation of the complexity of the mothers' role by healthcare professionals who attempt to work in partnership with mothers can mean they eventually can take the necessary risks in relinquishing their role of main carer for their ill/disabled adolescent. Caring for children with chronic conditions, thus, also means caring for mothers (Tong 2001).

Fathers' experiences

In the past a father's relationship with his child was considered as peripheral given that his main role was seen as to support the mother. However, current studies suggest that fathers play a much more important role in their child's development (Pelchat et al. 2003). For example, fathers and mothers display similar biologically-based reactions to babies (Schaffer 1994) and cross-cultural studies suggest that, when given the opportunity, fathers want to spend time with their offspring and can fulfil similar caretaking activities to that of mothers (Mackey 2001).

Fathers of chronically ill/disabled children not only share similar experiences as their partners, such as grieving for their 'well child' and for their previous family life, but also may, in many ways, perceive and respond to their child differently (West 2000; Waite-Jones and Madill 2008b). For example, parents often have different priorities: fathers stress the visibility of their child's condition and long-term future whilst mothers focus more on their child's ability to develop successful peer relationships and meet the challenges of daily living (Britton and Moore 2002).

Issues of masculinity

Fathers' gender identity and family role are also important, as having a disabled child can threaten a father's sense of masculinity through restricting his ability to act as the main, practical provider for his family (Chesler and Parry 2001). Despite new attitudes towards fatherhood (Baker and Lane 1994) and that potential challenges to masculinity through fathering a disabled child have been found to be countered by the fathers' sense of their increased importance within their family (Baumann and Braddick 1999), Chesler and Parry (2001) maintain that the concept of 'father as breadwinner' still permeates Western culture. Feeling judged against the traditional role of the man as provider can lead to a sense of incompetence for fathers struggling to protect their family, yet relegated to a supporting role due to the increased need for a division of labour in parenting (Sallfors and Hallberg 2003; Waite-Jones and Madill 2008b).

Ambivalent occupational constraints

Constraints of increased division of labour within parental roles experienced by fathers mean that they often work long hours to provide financially for their family whilst, most often, mothers undertake the main caretaking duties for their ill child. Baker and Lane (1994) found fathers to be more involved in child caretaking activities when mothers worked outside the home, but an ill child often leads to increased traditional division of labour with mothers most likely to be the partner giving up paid employment (Reay et al. 1998). Thus, whilst paid work may favour men in providing an identity and opportunity for self-worth outside their parenting role, fathers may not experience this as an active choice (Mac an Ghaill 1996; Connell 2002). Working outside the home also means fathers have less opportunity to be involved in the care of their ill/disabled child or shared social activities. Such restrictions compound the reduced 'playmate' role enjoyed by fathers of well children (Britton 2001; Sallfors and Hallberg 2003; Waite-Jones and Madill 2008b).

The level and type of engagement between fathers of an ill/disabled child will be determined by how masculinity and fatherhood are socially defined and reflected within social institutions (Chesler and Parry 2001). Bronfenbrenner's (1979: 2005) bio-ecological approach, referred to previously in Chapter 3, again illustrates how the fathers' role within his family is influenced by wider social forces, as values and beliefs of the macro-system underpin policies and practices of other systems impacting upon family life. Concepts of masculinity, embedded within Western society include physical and emotional resilience, with little concern for domestic chores and childcare (Connell 2002; Robertson 2006).

Emotional challenges

The emotional impact of having an ill/disabled child may expose fathers as vulnerable (Courtenay 2000; Seidler 2007) given that instru-mental (functional and active) behaviour is expected of men, whilst expressive (emotional and supportive) behaviour is considered femi-nine (Connell 1995). Fathers can be particularly conscious of their child's physical limitations, particularly those of a son, and miss out on shared sporting activities (Sallfors and Hallberg 2003; Waite-Jones and Madill 2008a). Sport provides shared social opportunities for fathers and sons enhancing (Connell 1995; Robertson 2006), reinforc-ing sons' development of a masculine identity (Watson 2000), and can contribute to 'male bonding' (Seidler 2007).

Given that current concepts of masculinity subordinate less powerful males, including those who are disabled (Courtenay 2000), fathers' sense of masculinity may be further threatened by a sense of fathering an ill/disabled child (Gerschick and Miller 2004). Thus, not only may fathers experience the loss of their 'ideal' child (Britton and Moore 2002; Waite-Jones and Madill 2008b) they may also feel a sense of personal and parental failure (Reay et al. 1998).

Whilst caring deeply for their ill/disabled child, fathers can also feel resentful of having less time to spend with their partner (Britton and Moore 2002; Waite-Jones and Madill 2008b). Fathers often conceal their emotions in an attempt to preserve their sense of masculinity and avoid burdening their family. However, this can also mean fathers concealing the true depth of their emotions from themselves (Seidler 2007).

Coping strategies

Fathers attempt to limit the impact of their distress through use of distraction and denial. Whilst work, which restricts involvement with the ill child, can be seen as fathers' way of caring for their families (Morgan 1992), it can also offer a distraction and fathers can feel guilty that this is not always an option for mothers (Sallfors and Hallberg 2003; Waite-Jones and Madill 2008b). Moreover, denial can be difficult to sustain for fathers who are constantly faced with the visibility of their child's condition (Baumann and Braddick 1999; Britton and Moore 2002; Waite-Jones and Madill 2008b). This may help to explain their reluctance to be involved in their child's hospital visits as these demand engagement with medical realities (Waite-Jones and Madill 2008b). Also, distraction and denial offer only short-term benefits and might delay adjustment to a chronic situation and problem-focused coping be ultimately more useful (West 2000).

That fathers conceal their anxiety may also help explain a paradox emerging in relation to experiences reported by parents of their interactions with healthcare professionals. Mothers often report that, despite fathers taking a peripheral caretaking role, their opinion was often more likely to be believed by healthcare professionals (see also Britton 2001; Waite-Jones and Madill 2008b). It may well be that fathers' attempts to conceal their true concerns, as well as reticence to become unpopular with healthcare professionals if they raise difficult issues (see also McNeill 2004), means that they do not appear as anxious as mothers (Waite-Jones and Madill 2008b). This may make fathers seem more credible to healthcare staff than do the mothers, particularly as this reinforces gender-based expectations of the 'rational' male and the 'emotional' female.

However, concealment can create further tensions for fathers as concealing their feelings to protect their partner, who is usually their most valued form of emotional support, can create difficulties in adjusting to having a child with a chronic condition (see also McNeill 2004). This concealing can often lead to conflict within relationships between partners as concealment, denial and distraction used by fathers can be misinterpreted by mothers as a lack of interest or support (Britton and Moore 2002; Waite-Jones and Madill 2008b).

Fathers can receive some support from friends who give practical help or companionship in distracting activities. However, this is often in a less visible way than support experienced by mothers and often takes place within shared public space, such as the local pub or gym, or through telephone calls made for other specific purposes (Waite-Jones and Madill 2008b). Nevertheless, such opportunity for emotional expression still has to be conducted according to masculine codes, as male friends may feel uncomfortable if exposed to too much direct disclosure (Walker 2004).

The depth of fathers' response to having a child with a chronic condition is difficult to assess. However, there is a need to try and understand their position, particularly as previous research has tended to focus on mothers' reports and assumed that both parents have similar reactions. In fact, mothers are not always aware of the fathers' experiences (Britton and Moore 2002; Waite-Jones and Madill 2008b).

Role restrictions created through providing care for a chronically ill/disabled child may create barriers for fathers' involvement with emotional aspects of family life. Thus, fathers' responses, as with those of other family members, have to be seen as dynamic and in relation to forces on, and within, the family.

Potential supporting role of grandparents

Children and their parents are also embedded in a wider, complex social group including relatives who offer care and can influence family dynamics. However, demographic changes within current British society, including more members of the same family surviving but less in each generation, means a more narrow, vertical family structure is emerging (Bernal and Anuncibay 2008). Such new, 'bean-pole' family structures and improved educational and employment experiences allow grandparents to play an increasingly supportive role within families (Smith 2005).

Clarke and Roberts (2003) found that grandparents provide practical, financial and emotional support. Whilst geographical proximity can determine the amount of practical assistance grandparents can offer the ill/disabled grandchild, siblings and parents, communication through telephone and the internet can mean they provide consistent emotional support. However, grandparents' age and socioeconomic position will also influence the type and amount of support they can give (Smith 2005).

Britton (2001) and Seagull (2000) stress the importance of grand-mothers in particular, as often playing a central role in the care of an ill/disabled child. However, grandfathers have also been found to be useful too (Clarke and Roberts 2003). The gender of the ill/disabled child is relevant in the ways grandparents become involved as grand-fathers may act as social companions for boys whilst grandmothers often accompany girls and boys on social events and hospital visits (Waite-Jones 2005).

Grandparents can provide stability during stressful family upheavals and also act as a confidant for older grandchildren (Smith 2005; Waite-Jones 2005) including the ill/disabled child. Some of the needs of well siblings can be met by grandparents, as even during their sibling's healthy periods, well children may still miss out as their parents try to catch up with other neglected duties (Spinetta and Deasy-Spinetta 1981).

Nevertheless, whilst grandparents generally benefit from their con-tributions to their grandchildren's care, too much involvement can prove stressful (Bernal and Anuncibay 2008). Thus, more needs to be known about grandparents' contributions to the care of children with chronic conditions, and how to support them too.

Chronic illness and disability across the family life-cycle

Given the family can be seen as a system, and having considered the impact of childhood chronic illness on different family members it can be seen that family life as a whole becomes medicalised with each member's life influenced, to some extent. Adverse social and emotional effects of having a chronic condition may intensify during late child-hood, with family members increasingly required to act as advocates and help ill/disabled adolescents to avoid social rejection and create an independent social life.

Mothers prove committed advocates given their emotional involve-ment in caring for their ill/disabled child and 'battle' on their behalf. However, this is often perceived as hyper-vigilance and contrasted to fathers' behaviour whose concern for their ill child is less overtly expressed as they conceal their feelings of loss and constraints in an attempt to protect their family. Whilst siblings, particularly those near in age, are in a good position to act as their ill brother or sister's advocate, their reactions are ambivalent due to their own position within family relationships. However, social support in terms of extended family, particularly grandparents, can help in adjusting to the demands of childhood chronic conditions on family life. Also, over time, these demands are assimilated into family life and, with increased maturity of the young person with the chronic condition and reduced external pressures such as those from the age-segregated, education system, families perceive themselves as less different to other families.

Nevertheless, wider financial and psychosocial demands created by chronic conditions strains family resources, reduces spontaneity of family activities, and risks fragmentation of family life due to less opportunities for shared activities (Britton and Moore 2002; Waite-Jones 2005). Moreover, there is a need to view a family's reaction, and adaptation to disability across the family life-cycle as adaptation has to be renegotiated at different times throughout the family life course in response to age and gender related behaviour of different family members (Sallfors and Hallberg 2003; Waite-Jones 2005).

Factors challenging or facilitating family adjustment can relate to family life-stage and structure as children with chronic conditions mature with observable milestones, particularly in relation to transition to secondary schooling, creating new challenges for them and their families (Britton and Moore 2002; Waite-Jones 2005).

Family structure is important as in two parent families there is greater polarisation of parental roles based on gender, and gender of the parent within single parent households can determine the type of emotional and physical care different parents can give. Sons and daughters with chronic conditions are likely to have close relationships with their mother if she took on the role of main carer. Fathers of daughters may continue their protective role and offer some physical care, whilst those of sons are less involved with their personal care and may find it harder to find a means of communicating with them. However, fathers eventually can find ways of establishing relationships through new, shared interests with their chronically ill/disabled son as they approach adulthood (Waite-Jones 2005).

The dynamic process of family relationships, heightened by medicalised experiences and influenced by gender roles and the particular family life-stage, can create situations, which, to some extent, are beyond the control of the individuals involved.

Helpful initiatives and interventions

Current attempts within healthcare to minimise disruption of family life for children with chronic conditions, by treating them through outpatient clinics wherever possible, means parents are faced with serious decisions regarding treatments and are heavily involved in the management of their child's condition. Whilst greater involvement can mean increased understanding and feelings of control, Southwood (1995: 3) points out that this 'is not without its costs, however, in terms of the time it requires and the drain it places on the family's emotional, physical and financial resources'. Maintaining management regimes, including regular medication and exercise programmes, can prove stressful for parents, as well as their ill child, and can also restrict physical activities for the whole family. A child with physical disabilities can thus be affected, not only by the condition and the debilitating limitations, but also by reactions of family members to the restrictions placed upon them.

Interactions with professionals can prove demanding for parents of children with an illness/disability, as a gap often exists between hospital and home services (Limbrick-Spencer 2000) and professionals from a number of agencies are encountered separately. For example, parents have to liaise with healthcare professionals, social services, schools and local educational authorities. The large number of appointments, clinics, therapy sessions, and home visits can be chaotic, taking energy and time with repeated assessments, interviews and reviews. These are usually coordinated by the mother who has to remember who has been told what. Such experiences can prove frustrating for parents who may be asked for the same information by different professionals who are unaware of other agencies involved (Limbrick 2001). In addition, such visits require considerable economic outlay from families, and involve other stresses such as transport and parking.

It is important for healthcare professionals to be aware of the constraints on family life and help families adapt to having an ill/disabled child, and develop skills that can only come with experience and over time. It will be particularly useful for professionals to recognise differences in parents' reactions and the extent to which mothers are forced into a vigilant role and fathers may be concealing their emotions. Greater effort could be made to include fathers more in the care of the child, which may mean educating mothers on fathers' reactions and enlisting their help in improving and maintaining contact.

Healthcare and other professionals would also benefit from greater awareness of the potentially emotionally charged nature of relationships between professionals and family members and how displacement of anxiety and frustration can potentially occur on both sides. There is also a need for improved communication between healthcare professionals and schools and appreciation of the importance of voluntary groups in offering a 'voice' for families, which may be useful within this process.

The influence of national policies and legislation

The need to support families is increasingly recognised at a national level, particularly as the cost of caring for a chronically ill/disabled child can be three times higher than that for a well child (Williams 2004). Much of the Children Act 1989, which stresses the responsibilities as well as rights of parents, underpins current child services and plans for further improvements (White et al. 1990). For example, the implementation of directives from the Green Paper *Every Child Matters* (DH/DfES 2005), the Children Act, 2004, the Childcare Act 2006 and the related *National Service Framework for Children, Young Persons and Maternity Services* (DH/DfES 2004), has produced new initiatives and integrated ways of supporting children and families, including their involvement in planning and delivery, with coordinated services and information sharing between agencies. Parents are ensured a stronger role in their child's education, schools are offering extended services and there is increased spending on the needs of adolescents.

Moreover, the need to care for carers has been formally recognised through legislation with the Carer (Equal Opportunities) Act 2004. This offers financial support and allows local authorities to address the needs of those with parental responsibility for a disabled child who provide, or intend to provide care, on a regular basis, and the Social Care Institute of for Excellence have established guidelines of good practice.

An even more recent government document, *Aiming High for Children: Supporting Families* (DH/DfES 2007) emphasises the importance of resilience building and offering personalised, proactive help for families. Integrated support for families with complex needs, including learning disabilities and physical disabilities, is recommended. However, whilst the need for specialist services is acknowledged, the introduction and exit plans required may not prove possible for children with lifelong conditions.

Nevertheless, packages of tailored help for families are advocated and recognition given to the need to support community groups and voluntary agencies as they, too, can play a valuable part in supporting such families. For example, national charities such as Banardo's offer workshops and activities for different family members and there is growing recognition within Arthritis Care that, whilst providing some excellent support for adults, even more work needs to be done to find ways of helping children, young people and their families (personal communication). Appropriate support depends upon the age of the child and their illness status, which means that very different, flexible forms of help are required. For instance, involvement with support groups are useful during flare-up periods, but can serve as unpleasant reminders during the child's well periods. Also, during adolescence and early adulthood young people may wish to have little connection to any organisation related to their condition, yet still need social support from others who truly understand.

Supportive interventions, thus, need to be appropriate for different stages across the family life-cycle. Parents/carers of very young children manage the social and educational life of their child but need supporting in this. Since 1998, the Government initiative Sure Start has included help for families of children with special needs at a pre-school level, but there is still a need for further consideration as to what constitutes effective support (Belsky et al. 2006). In contrast, adolescents with chronic conditions need support in achieving independence, whilst parents require support and understanding in relinquishing their skilled, advocate role.

McDonagh et al. (2000) point out the complex legal position in which parents and healthcare professionals are placed in relation to caring for children as they develop. The Children Act 1989 stresses parental duties, rather than rights, but also that a child under 16 years of age, if deemed 'competent', can make decisions about their own treatment and care. Paradoxically children under 16 years also cannot legally refuse treatment. McDonagh et al. (2000) explain how important consent is for compliance, and that compromise is often the only option.

Healthcare provision, thus, also needs to be appropriate for the developmental stages of children and adolescents as they move from paediatric to adult services. McDonagh (2007: 803) suggests that 'transition is an age and developmentally appropriate process, addressing the psycho-social and educational/vocational aspects of care in addition to the traditional medical areas', and that the planning for this event should start from the day of diagnosis. However, understanding, education and training is needed for families, staff and the young person, for adolescents to confidently interact with professionals without parent/carer presence.

As the views of professionals and parents are not always compatible sensitivity and understanding is required to support parents as they relinquish their role of expert, advocates. Watson et al. (2002) suggest a transdisciplinary team approach, including the family, transferring skills and knowledge and developing a sense of trust.

The importance of information and education

To develop such a good team relationships within healthcare means keeping family members informed and educating them about psychosocial aspects, as well as physical elements of the child/young person's condition. Patient education and other educational interventions have been seen as useful in relation to a number of chronic conditions and disorders including autism, mental health and learning disability (Lobato and Kao 2002; Williams et al. 2003).

However, Barlow and Ellard's (2004) review of existing literature on psychosocial educational interventions suggests that much more help is needed, particularly for parents and siblings. They found that existing interventions tend to focus on management of the condition (particularly in relation to asthma and diabetes) with little attention given to psychosocial issues. However, cognitive behavioural type interventions (CBT was discussed in detail in Chapter 3) were found to be useful in terms of helping improve self-efficacy, self-management, pain control and social competence in the young person and overall family function.

However, timing of information may be important as Barlow and Ellard (2004) identified particular vulnerable periods in the trajectory of children's experiences of chronic conditions, such as when a diagnosis is given. The particular vulnerability of siblings during adolescence suggests a need to seek further understanding of appropriate support which can be offered at such times, particularly for those who do not receive it from the extended family. More services are, thus, needed to help empower and improve self-care in adolescent and support their parents and other family members.

Within this chapter it has not been possible to do justice to the diverse experiences of specific childhood conditions, family types and structures or ethnic groups. However, whilst these issues need further, serious consideration an attempt has been made to try and distil evidence of some shared experiences, and offer some indication of the impact of childhood chronic conditions on children and their families.

Conclusion

An attempt has been made within this chapter to convey the importance of recognising the impact of childhood chronic conditions on the whole family, and in particular:

- possible psychological and social consequences of having a chronic condition, including altered body image, difficult peer relationships, and increased dependence on family members to attain independence
- potential amplification of ambivalent relationships between siblings and their ill/disabled brother or sister, and impact on well sibling's own social relationships
- the need for greater understanding of the position of mothers as expert knowledge holders and vigilant advocates of their ill child, as this may be misperceived as over-protectiveness
- the extent to which fathers may conceal their emotional responses to having an ill/disabled child, and use of distraction and denial as coping strategies, which may be misunderstood as lack of concern and create family friction
- increasing recognition of the role of extended family members, especially grandparents, in supporting children with chronic conditions and their family
- how family structure, birth order of siblings and gendered relationships of family members, have to be considered to appreciate the complexity of family adjustment to the child/adolescent's condition, at different points of the family life-cycle
- increasing recognition of the needs of the whole family and appropriate support within current legislation as well as policies and initiatives within healthcare and the voluntary sector.

References

Anthony K.E., Gill M. and Schanberg E. (2003) Brief report: Parental perceptions of child vulnerability in children with chronic illness. *Journal of Paediatric Psychology* 28: 185–90.

Arkela-Kautianen M., Haapasaari J., Kautianenen H., Vilkkumaa I., Malkia W. and Leirislalo-Repo M. (2005) Favourable social functioning and health related quality of life of patients with JIA in early adulthood. *Annals of Rheumatic Diseases* 64: 875–80.

Baker S. and Lane M. (1994) The good father. *Child Health* 2: 28–30.

Baraitser L. and Noack A. (2007) Mother Courage: reflections on maternal resilience. *British Journal of Psychotherapy* 23(2): 171–88.

Barlow J.H. and Ellard D.R. (2004) Psycho-educational interventions for children with chronic disease, parents and siblings: an overview of the research evidence base. *Child: Care, Health and Development* 30: 637–45.

Barlow J.H., Harrison K. and Shaw K. (1998) The experience of parenting in the context of juvenile chronic arthritis. *Clinical Child Psychology and Psychiatry* 3(3): 445–63.

Barlow J.H., Wright C.C., Shaw K.L., Luqman R. and Wyness I.J. (2002) Maternal stressors, maternal well being and children's well being in the context of juvenile idiopathic arthritis. *Early Child Development and Care* 172(1): 89–98.

Batte S., Watson A.R. and Amess K. (2006) The effects of chronic renal failure on siblings. *Paediatric Nephrology* 21: 246–50.

Baumann S.L. and Braddick M. (1999) Out of their element: fathers of children who are 'not the same'. *Journal of Pediatric Nursing* 14(6): 369–78.

Beattie P.E. and Lewis-Jones M.S. (2006) A comparative study of impairment of quality of life in children with skin disease and children with other chronic childhood diseases. *British Journal of Dermatology* 155(1): 145–51.

Belsky J., Melhuish E., Barnes J., Leyland A.H. and Romaniuk J. (2006) Effects of Sure Start local programmes on children and families: early findings from a quasi-experimental, cross sectional study. *British Medical Journal*, www.bmj.com.wam.leeds.aac.uk/cgi/content/full/332/7556/1476?maxtoshow= . . . (accessed 17 January 2007).

Bennett T., DeLuca A. and Allen R. (1996) Families of children with disabilities: positive adaptation across the life cycle. *Social Work in Education* 18(1): 31–44.

Bernal J.G. and de la Fuente Anucibay R. (2008) Intergenerational grandparent/grandchild relations: the socioeducational role of grandparents. *Educational Gerontology* 34: 67–88.

Billings G., Moos R.H., Miller J.J. and Gottleib J.E. (1987) Psychosocial adaptation in juvenile rheumatic disease: a controlled evaluation. *Health Psychology* 6(4): 343–59.

Bradford R. (1997) *Children, Families and Chronic Disease*. London: Routledge.

Britton C. (2001) *Telling It How It Is*. Birmingham: Hanseltrust Publications.

Britton C. and Moore A. (2002) Views from the inside, Part 2: What the children with ARTHRITIS said, and the experiences of siblings, mothers, fathers and grandparents. *British Journal of Occupational Therapy* 65(9): 413–19.

Bronfenbrenner U. (1979) *The Ecology of Human Development: Experiments by the nature and design*. Cambridge, Mass: Harvard University Press.

Bronfenbrenner U. (2005) *Making Human Beings Human: Bioecological perspectives on human development*. Thousand Oaks, CA: Sage Publications.

Burman E. (1995) *Deconstructing Developmental Psychology*. London: Routledge.

Bywater P., Ali Z., Fazil Q., Wallace L.M. and Singh G. (2003) Attitudes towards disability amongst Pakistani and Bangladeshi parents of disabled children in the UK: considerations fro service providers and the disability movement. *Health and Social Care in the Community* 11(6): 502–9.

Chesler M.A. and Parry C. (2001) Gender roles and/or styles in crisis: an integrative analysis of the experiences of fathers of children with cancer. *Qualitative Health Research* 11: 363–84.

Clarke L. and Roberts G. (2003) Grandparenthood: Its Meaning and Its Contribution to Older People's Lives. G0 Findings 22. ESRC Growing Older Programme. Sheffield: University of Sheffield, pp. 1–4.

Connell R.W. (1995) *Masculinities*. Cambridge: Polity Press.

Connell R.W. (2002) *Gender*. Cambridge: Polity Press.

Courtenay W.H. (2000) Constructions of masculinity and their influence on men's well-being: a theory of gender and health. *Social Science and Medicine* 50: 1385–401.

Cunningham-Burley S., Beckett-Milburn K. and Kemmer D. (2006) Constructing health and sickness in the context of motherhood and paid work. *Sociology of Health and Illness* 28(4): 385–409.

Dahlquist L.M. (2003) Are children with JRA and their families at risk or resilient? *Journal of Pediatric Psychology* 28(1): 45–6.

Dallos R. and Draper R. (2006) *An Introduction to Family Therapy. Systemic Theory and Practice*. Maidenhead: Berkshire.

Daniel E., Ken G., Binney V. and Pagdin J. (2005) Trying to do my best, as a mother: decision-making in families of children undergoing elective surgical treatment for short stature. *British Journal of Health Psychology* 10(1): 101–14.

Department of Health and Department for Education and Skills (DH/DfES) (2004) *The National Service Framework for Children, Young People and Maternity Services*. London: The Stationery Office.

Department of Health and Department for Education and Skills (DH/DfES) (2005) *Every Child Matters*. London: The Stationery Office.

Department of Health and Department for Education and Skills (DH/DfES) (2007) *Aiming High for Children: Supporting Families*. London: The Stationery Office.

Dixon-Wood M. (2007) Childhood cancer as a chronic illness. *Chronic Illness* 3: 251–2.

Dunn J. (2000) State of the art: siblings. *The Psychologist* 13(5): 244–8.

Edwards M. and Davis H. (1997) *Counselling Children with Chronic Medical Conditions*. Leicester: BPS Books.

Gerhardt C.A., Vannatta K., McKellop M., Taylor J., Passo M., Reiter-Purtill J., Zeller M. and Noll R.B. (2003) Brief Report: Child-rearing practices of caregivers with and without a child with juvenile rheumatoid arthritis: perspectives of caregivers and professionals. *Journal of Pediatric Psychology* 28(4): 275–9.

Gerschick T.J. and Miller A.S. (2004) Coming to terms with masculinity and physical disability. In: M.S. Kimmel and M.A. Messner (eds) *Men's Lives*. London: Pearson Education, pp. 349–62.

Gittins D. (1993) *The Family in Question*. London: Macmillan.

Guell C. (2007) Painful childhood: children living with juvenile arthritis. *Qualitative Health Research* 17(7): 884–92.

Harding R. (1996) Children with cancer: the needs of siblings. *Professional Nurse* 11(9): 588–90.

Hockney J. and James A. (2003) *Social Identities Across the Life Course.* Basingstoke: Palgrave Macmillan.

Houtzager B.A., Oort F.J., Hoekstra-Weebers J.E.H.M., Caron H.N., Grootenhuis M.A. and Last B.F. (2004) Coping and family functioning predict longitudinal psychological adaptation of siblings of childhood cancer patients. *Journal of Pediatric Psychology* 29(8): 591–605.

Huygen A.C., Kuis W. and Sinnema G. (2000) Psychological, behavioural, and social adjustment in children and adolescents with juvenile chronic arthritis. *Annals of the Rheumatic Diseases* 59: 2776–282.

Kashikar-Zuck, Lynch A.M., Graham T.B., Swain N.F., Mullen S.M. and Noll R.B. (2007) Social functioning and peer relationships of adolescents with juvenile fibromyalgia syndrome. *Arthritis and Rheum* 57(3): 474–80.

Krulik T. and Florian V. (1995) Social isolation of school-age children with chronic illnesses. *Social Sciences and Health* 1(3): 164–74.

Laxer R.M. (1999) Long-term toxicity of immune suppression in juvenile rheumatic diseases. *Rheumatology* 38: 1743–6.

LeBovidge J.S., Lavigne J.V., Donenberg G. and Miller M.L. (2003) Psychological adjustment of children and adolescents with chronic arthritis: a meta-analytic review. *Journal of Pediatric Psychology* 28(1): 29–39.

Limbrick P. (2001) *The Team Around the Child.* Manchester: Interconnections.

Limbrick-Spencer G. (2000) *Parents' Support Needs.* Birmingham: Hanseltrust Publications.

Lobato D.J. and Kao B.T. (2002) Integrated sibling–parent group intervention to improve sibling knowledge and adjustment to chronic illness and disability. *Journal of Pediatric Psychology* 27(8): 711–16.

Lustig J.L., Ireys H.T., Sills E.M. and Walsh B.B. (1996) Mental health of mothers of children with juvenile rheumatoid arthritis: appraisal as a mediator. *Journal of Pediatric Psychology* 21: 719–33.

Mac an Ghaill M. (1996) *Understanding Masculinities.* Buckingham: Open University Press.

Mackey W.C. (2001) Support for the existence of an independent man-to-child affiliative bond: fatherhood as a biocultural invention. *Psychology of Men and Masculinity* 2: 51–66.

MacLeod K. (1995) A Study of the Social, Emotional and Practical needs of Children with Juvenile Chronic Arthritis and their Families. Publication for the Lady Hoare Trust based on unpublished PhD thesis, pp. 1–12.

Manuel J. (2001) Risk and resistance factors in the adaptation in mothers of children with juvenile rheumatoid arthritis. *Journal of Pediatric Psychology* 26(4): 237–46.

McDonagh J.E. (2007) Transition of care fro paediatric to adult rheumatology. *Archives of Diseases of Children* 92: 802–7.

McDonagh J.E., Southwood T.R. and Ryder C.A. (2000) Bridging the gap in rheumatology. *Annals of Rheumatology Diseases* 59: 86–93.

McNeill T. (2004) Fathers' experience of parenting a child with juvenile rheumatoid arthritis. *Qualitative Health Research* 14(4): 526–45.

Mescon J.A. and Honig A.S. (1995) Parents, teachers and medical personnel: helping children with chronic illness. *Child Development and Care* 111: 107–29.

Miller S. (1996) Living with a disabled sibling. *Paediatric Nursing* 8(8): 21–4.

Morgan D.H.J. (1992) *Discovering Men.* London: Routledge.

Pelchat D., Lefebvre H. and Perreault M. (2003) Differences and similarities between mothers' and fathers' experiences of parenting a child with a disability. *Journal of Child Health Care* 7: 231–47.

Peterson L.S., Mason T., Nelson A.M., O'Fallon W.M. and Gabriel S. (1997) Psychosocial outcomes and health status of adults who have had juvenile rheumatoid arthritis. *Arthritis and Rheumatism* 40(12): 2235–40.

Power T.G., Dahlquist L.M., Thompson S.M. and Warren R. (2003) Interactions between children with juvenile rheumatoid arthritis and their mothers. *Journal of Pediatric Psychology* 28: 213–21.

Price B. (1993) Diseases and altered body image in children. *Paediatric Nursing* 5(6): 18–21.

Ratcliffe J. (2001) *Listening to siblings.* Birmingham: Hanseltrust Publications.

Reay D., Bignold S., Ball S.J. and Cribb A. (1998) 'He just had a different way of showing it': Gender dynamics in families coping with childhood cancer. *Journal of Gender Studies* 7: 39–52.

Reiter-Purtill J., Gerhardt C., Vannatta K., Passo M.H. and Noll R.B. (2003) A controlled longitudinal study of the social functioning of children with juvenile rheumatoid arthritis. *Journal of Pediatric Psychology* 28: 17–28.

Robertson S. (2006) 'I've been like a coiled spring this last week': Embodied masculinity and health. *Sociology of Health and Illness* 28: 433–56.

Sallfors C. and Hallberg L.R-M. (2003) A parental perspective on living with a chronically ill child: a qualitative study. *Family Systems and Health* 21(2): 193–203.

Sallfors C., Fasth A. and Halberg L.R-M. (2002) Oscillating between hope and despair – a qualitative study. *Child: Care, Health and Development* 28(6): 495–505.

Sandstrom M.J. and Schonberg L.E. (2004) Brief Report: Peer rejection, social behaviour, and psychological adjustment in children with juvenile rheumatic disease. *Journal of Pediatric Psychology* 29(1): 29–34.

Schafer M., Korn S., Smith P.K., Hunter S.C., Mora-Merchan J.A., Singer M.M. and van der Meulen K. (2004) Lonely in the crowd: recollections of bullying. *British Journal of Developmental Psychology* 22: 379–94.

Schaffer H.R. (1994) *Making Decisions about Children.* Oxford: Blackwell.

Schanberg L.E., Anthony K.K., Gil K.M., Lefebvre J.C., Kredich D.W. and Marcharoni L.M. (2001) Family pain history predicts child health status in children with chronic rheumatic disease. *Pediatrics* 108 (3): http://www.pediatrics.org/cgi/content/full/108/3/e47 (accessed 28 Feb 2007).

Seagull E.A. (2000) Beyond mothers and children: Finding the Family I. Pediatric psychology. *Journal of Pediatric Psychology* 25(3): 161–9.

Seidler V.J. (2007) Masculinities, bodies and emotional life. *Men and Masculinities* 10: 9–12.

Sharpe D. and Rossiter L. (2002) Siblings of children with a chronic illness: a meta-analysis. *Journal of Pediatric Psychology* 27(8): 699–710.

Silver E.J. and Frohlinger-Graham M.J. (2000) Brief Report: Psychological symptoms in healthy female siblings of adolescents with and without chronic conditions. *Journal of Pediatric Psychology* 25(4): 279–84.

Sloper P. (2000) Experiences and support needs of siblings of children with cancer. *Health and Social care in the Community* 8: 298–306.

Smith P.K. (2005) Grandparents and Grandchildren. *The Psychologist* 18(11): 684–7.

Southwood T. (1995) *Forward to Living with Juvenile Chronic Arthritis.* Arthritis Research Council Publication.

Spinetta J. (1981) *The sibling of the child with cancer.* In: J. Spinetta and P. Deasy-Spinetta (eds) *Living with Childhood Cancer.* Mosby: St Louis, 133–42.

Straughair S. (1992) *The Experiences of Young People with Arthritis.* London: Joseph Rowntree Foundation, pp. 26–9.

Sturge C., Garralda M.E., Boissin M., Dore C.J. and Woo P. (1997) School attendance and juvenile chronic arthritis. *British Journal of Rheumatology* 36: 1218–23.

Tong R. (2001) Just caring about women's and children's health: some feminist perspectives. *Journal of Medicine and Philosophy* 26(2): 147–62.

Upton P. and Eiser C. (2006) School experiences after treatment for brain tumour. *Child Care, Health and Development* 32(1): 9–17.

von Weiss R.T., Rapoff M.A., Varni J.W., Lindsley C.B., Olson N.Y., Madson K.L. and Bernstein B.H. (2002) Daily hassles and social support as predictors of adjustment in children with pediatric rheumatic disease. *Journal of Pediatric Psychology* 27(2): 155–65.

Waite-Jones J.M. (2005) Juvenile Arthritis and Family Function. University of Leeds: Unpublished PhD thesis.

Waite-Jones J.M. and Madill A. (2008a) Amplified ambivalence: having a sibling with juvenile idiopathic arthritis. *Psychology and Health* 23(4): 477–92.

Waite-Jones J.M. and Madill A. (2008b) Concealed concern: experiences of having a child with juvenile idiopathic arthritis. *Psychology and Health* In press.

Walker K. (2004) 'I'm not friends the way she's friends': ideological and behavioural constructions of masculinity in men's friendships. In M.S. Kimmel and M.A. Messner (eds) *Men's Lives.* London: Pearson Education, pp. 389–401.

Wallander J.L. and Varni J.W. (1998) Effects of pediatric chronic physical disorders on child and family adjustment. *Journal of Child Psychology* 39(1): 29–46.

Watson D., Townsley R., Abbott D. and Latham P. (2002) *Working Together*. Birmingham: Handseltrust Publications.

Watson J. (2000) *Male Bodies*. Buckingham: Open University Press.

West S. (2000) *Just a Shadow: A review of support for fathers of children with disabilities*. Birmingham: Hanseltrust Publications.

White P.H. (1996) Future expectations: Adolescents with rheumatic diseases and their transition into adulthood. *British Journal of Rheumatology* 35: 80–3.

White R., Carr P. and Low N. (1990) *A Guide to the Children Act 1989*. London: Butterworth.

Williams C. (2002) *Mothers, Young People and Chronic Illness*. Hampshire: Ashgate Publishing Ltd.

Williams F. (2004) *Rethinking Families*. London: Calouste Gullenkian Foundation.

Williams P.D., Williams A.R., Graff J.C., Hanson S., Stanton A., Hafeman C., Liebeergen A., Leuenberg K., Setter R.K., Ridder L., Curry H., Barnard M. and Sanders S. (2003) A community-based intervention for siblings and parents of children with a chronic illness or disability: the ISEE study. *Journal of Pediatrics* 143: 386–93.

Woo P. and Wedderburn L.R. (1998) Juvenile chronic arthritis. *Lancet* I(351): 969–73.

Yantzi N.M., Rosenberg M.W. and McKeever P. (2006) Getting out of the house: the challenges mothers face when their children have long-term care needs. *Health and Social Care in the Community* 15(1): 45–55.

Chapter 9

Challenges and acts of creation faced by health professionals

Jo Gilmartin

In the exploration of health psychology, we have travelled a very long way; many magnificent themes have been examined. The premise of this chapter is that, in the treatment of psychological processes affecting the individual health experience, changing health behaviour has a specific contribution to make. In the case of body image dissatisfaction or severe obesity the patient's relationship with food or self-conception may be understood more fully by deconstructing beliefs systems. It is vital, then, to see the situation in its true light. The reconstruction of beliefs requires more than a paradigmatic change. The challenge for health professionals is not only tackling resistance when circumstances are not propitious but also being aware of their own emotional well-being and intention. This chapter, then, is concerned with the challenge of changing self-limiting beliefs, the embodiment of the health practitioner intention, the centrality of energy psychology and the usefulness of evidence-based practice (EBP).

Paradigmatic change in beliefs

There are several theories that offer legitimate and optimistic interventions for changing health beliefs and health behaviour (Conner and Norman 2005; Kerr et al. 2005). A consideration of some psychological interventions currently available such as CBT and family therapy is presented in Chapters 3, 4, 5 and 6. Nonetheless, changing health

beliefs is often threatening. People troubled by body image dissatisfaction and plagued by obesity or eating disorders might have deep
feelings of helplessness in controlling significant areas of their lives.
Furthermore, they might embrace Darwin's version of evolution regarding hereditary genes passed on from parents, impacting on the control
of obesity characteristics, emotion and behaviour. This type of thinking
can foster a belief of victimhood and impotence, which can be debilitating. Lipton's (2005) revolutionary work on the biology of belief and
epigenetics is today a very active area of scientific research. Although
beyond the scope of this chapter, it is a powerful source in regard to
shedding light on gene activity.

Despite the challenges and resistance portrayed by patients, health
professionals need to facilitate change with clarity and positive
intention. To help service users shift beliefs and accomplish goals,
evidence-based practice, energy psychology techniques and internet
information might be useful. Firstly, it is crucial to explore evidenced-
based practice because it has the potential to bring a greater enrich-
ment to care practice.

Evidence-based practice

Glimpses of ways of empowering patients to change health beliefs can
be gained from evidence-based practice. Evidence-based intervention
sets the tone in healthcare and has important implications for changing
health behaviour and patient outcomes. Increasingly, practitioners are
being positioned in active decision-making roles by policy makers and
the government modernisation agenda (Ring et al. 2006). Of great
significance, then, is what counts as research evidence: knowing the
patient, including typical preferences, the clinical knowledge and
expertise of the health professional, contextual resources (Thompson
et al. 2004) and cultural variables. This process requires 'active engagement by health professionals in terms of accessing, appraising, and
incorporating research evidence into their practice' (Thompson et al.
2004: 68). Although the evidence-based practice (EBP) paradigm is
attractive in the power that it gives practitioners over disease and suffering (Grypdonck 2006: 1374), nonetheless, it renders many issues
objective and controllable. Therefore, a major challenge for health
professionals is critical appraisal and the employment of choice in the
utilisation of evidence.

Evidence-based practice has become a growth industry and its evolution has given birth to inspirational resources such as the Cochrane
Collaboration, clinical protocols and a range of journals (*Evidence-*

Based Nursing, Evidence-Based Medicine). The National Institute for Health and Clinical Excellence (NICE) has been set up to encourage its development, although there is much controversy about its uptake and utilisation. Upton and Upton (2005) reported that national initiatives had a positive impact on nurses' attitudes towards clinical effectiveness. However, influencing behaviour appears to be more troublesome due to the lack of required skills, time and the burden of clinical work. Thompson and Dowding (2002) point to knowledge-based deficits that impact on decision-making including overconfidence or over-reliance on experiential knowledge.

Changing and shaping health behaviour

Unsurprisingly, health psychologists concerned with behaviour change prefer to focus on efficacy questions because their interest lies in change processes and health outcomes. However, according to Wardle and Steptoe (2005: 674) this approach might restrict data analysis to the participants who adhere to protocol and attended for follow-up, perhaps excluding those who dropped out. This design could be problematic because effectiveness of an intervention might be overestimated with dilution of efficacy estimates. Steptoe (2004) points to randomised controlled trials (RCT) displaying favourable effects of physical activity for depression in comparison with control procedures but the dropout rates were substantial. This could possibly lead to a false impression of the benefits of a programme if generalised to the whole population. Thus methodological rigour with the intention-to-treat-analysis (participants remain in the analysis even if they drop out of the study) is vital to build up a strong evidence base.

Despite the number of large-scale psychological driven intervention studies currently available, for example, Berkman et al.'s (2003) randomised trial of cognitive behavioural treatment of depression following a myocardial infarction, health professionals facing the challenge of changing health behaviour will need to embrace rigorous research and sound decision-making. This will involve the interplay of factors and processes (Thompson 2003) that underpin EBP. The process is often complex because of competing interests, value conflicts and experiential knowledge among multidisciplinary team members.

Different types of information influence the process, including protocols, and research evidence, the experiential knowledge of health professionals, the patients' attitude, motivation and preference, and cultural and local contextual variables. For example, in the case of employing interventions to reduce obesity a perspective that goes beyond individuals' needs is crucial. Wardle and Steptoe (2005: 674) forefront research approaches that address 'casual associations between environmental change and health change', thus emphasising the need to develop 'health promoting' environments as an important variable in tackling population trends in obesity. The major challenge is perhaps how these influences are weighted and integrated to achieve a positive outcome for the patient.

In addition, when research questions extend beyond the effectiveness of an intervention and might include, for example, underlying psycho-social concerns regarding 'body dissatisfaction', multiple factors might influence determining the best evidence (http://www.cebm.net/levels_of_evidence.asp). The trajectory towards intervention choice will have aspirations for effectiveness, appropriateness and feasibility. Further-more, as Evans (2003) points out, evidence on the latter three dimen-sions can have significant effects for evaluating health care interventions. Crucially, health professionals need to recognise the range of dimen-sions that evidence should address before they can be adequately appraised. Despite the usefulness of hierarchies of evidence for ranking purposes, they only provide a guide in terms of the strength of the avail-able evidence; the quality of the research is also a major influence.

Because of the strong contemporary association between research protocols/national guidelines and clinical effectiveness, scholarly dis-cussion deals with the uptake of guidelines. This trend is demonstrated in a recent study undertaken by Bryer (2006), reporting that junior rheumatology nurses appear to blend influencing factors competently in two inpatient rheumatology wards in the north of England. Interest-ingly, the nurses appeared to use locally produced guidelines and clinical nurse specialists for information, veering away from the imple-mentation of new research findings. Implementing national guidelines and new research into practice requires more than a focus on individ-ual health professionals but requires the commitment of teams and organisations.

Sheldon et al. (2004) highlight significant organisational features, for instance, a culture of consensus, financial stability and a strong governance function, which were giving birth to an absorptive capacity for national guidelines and new research. The challenge is to create organisations with these capacities, given the economic and political constraints that prevail in the health care systems. Nonetheless, if healthcare professionals are expected to utilise national guidelines and EBP effectively, resources need to be invested in encouraging and enabling them with this huge undertaking. This is vital as health professionals try to disrupt some of the ways in which people have come to believe and think about toxic health and well-being.

Furthermore practitioners should aim to decouple the link between health and passivity, or at least decentre it, by positing alternative explanations such as the link between weight loss and physical activity or self-enhancement and body satisfaction.

Energy psychology

There is an interesting twist in the concrete argument of scientific enlightenment in this post-modern area; some service users 'react against science', viewing evidence-based practice with suspicion, thus provocatively giving birth to a new enthusiasm for energy medicine and complementary therapies. There is an increasing interest in understanding how complementary and alternative medicine influence healing and promote well-being. These are vitally important issues, with renowned critiques emerging including the striking investigation and appraisal put forward by Adams (2007) and Adams and Tovey (2008).

The same is true for energy psychology because the energy body holds the blueprint, 'the infrastructure, the invisible foundation for the health of the body' (Feinstein et al. 2005: 2). The body is composed of energy centres that interplay dynamically with thoughts, moods, organs and cells. The subtle energies include electromagnetic impulses, which can be recorded by a magnetic resonance imaging (MRI) or electroencephalography (EEG). Energy psychology builds on established psychological principles such as conditioned response in human activity and the impact of early experience on current emotional and behaviour patterns (Feinstein et al. 2005).

Moreover, energy psychology also has a specific role to play. This involves stimulating energy points on the skin which, paired with specified mental activities, can instantly shift the brain's electrochemistry; for instance, to help a client change unwanted eating or smoking habits and behaviour and help overcome unwanted emotions such as guilt, fear, anxiety, shame, anger or jealously. Changing health behaviour, then, has a kind of ecology, in which a variety of types of interaction merge into one another, and there is a continuing succession. The challenge for the health professional is to create an atmosphere where clients are able to deal with conflict, change, frustration, loss, growth, transition and empowerment. Energy psychology offers a serious and sustained attempt to dramatically enhance changing health behaviour. The innovative process helps clients shift problematic beliefs, behaviour and emotions with 'a precision and gentleness that is unprecedented within psychotherapy' (Feinstein et al. 2005: 2).

Energy psychology applies principles and techniques for working with the body's physical energy to facilitate changes in thoughts, emotions and behaviour. There are numerous specific formulations such as emotional freedom techniques (Look 2005), thought field therapy (Callahan 2001), Tapas acupressure technique (www.unstressforsuccess.com) and eye movement desensitisation and reprocessing (EMDR). The body is 'a cascading fountain of energy systems, exquisitely coordinated, and entirely unique' (Eden 2007: 29). Energy psychology works predominantly with the meridians used in acupuncture, acknowledged by modern scientists too (O'Becker 1985). The meridians appear to be an interface between the physical body and the etheric body, being the innermost layer of the human energy field (Gerber 2001).

Forms of emotional distress or physical symptoms are a disruption to the body's energy system. Energy might be blocked, scrambled, weak or not flowing properly, frequently experienced as negative emotion or physical symptoms. Self-esteem threats experienced by women's exposure to thin media images often lead to body image dissatisfaction, 'when favourable views about oneself are questioned, impugned, mocked, or otherwise challenged' (Jarry 2007: 40). Self-loathing and negative emotions that are recycled short-circuit energy systems and are a salient source of self-esteem problems. Energy psychology helps people break through unworthiness, judgement, anxiety, guilt, shame and egotistical fear, promoting harmony, well-being and coherence.

Tapping directions

The most popular form is emotional freedom technique (EFT), which involves tapping on specific meridians while focusing on a troublesome emotion, issue or symptom. The basic self-help method can be learned fairly quickly but skill and sophistication is required for complex issues. In some instances underlying emotional drivers such as traumatic memories, feelings associated with addictions or self-defeating habits or dysfunctional beliefs might require in–depth exploration. For instance, in cases of obesity exploring eating behaviour including cravings and associated feeling states is important. Although still considered experimental, these techniques are being used by therapists, nurses, physicians and lay people globally (Look 2005).

The first step in using EFT involves pairing the troublesome emotion or symptom with an expression of self-acceptance and self-worth. For example, 'Even though I feel fat and hopeless about losing weight, I

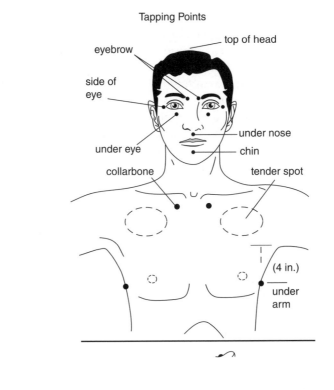

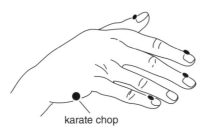

Figure 9.1 EFT tapping points. Source: Arenson (2001) designed by Laurence Brockway.

deeply and completely accept myself', 'Even though I feel anxious in my stomach when I think about coping alone with the arthritis, I choose to accept myself completely and feel relaxed about it right now'. Then you proceed to tap on the eight EFT acupoints sharply (Figure 9.1), while focusing on the setup statement. Tapping can be done with either hand or with both hands simultaneously. The fingertips of your index finger and middle finger can facilitate tapping effectively, or perhaps make a 'three-finger notch' by including your thumb.

Look (2005) suggests starting at the inner eyebrow point; begin tapping each point in the sequence approximately 7 to 10 times while repeating the setup phrase provided for the specific issue: side of the eye, under eye, under nose, indent of chin, immediately below the inner end of collar-bone, under arm (aligned with nipples), and top of head.

Two rounds of positive tapping sequence can follow this. Starting at the inner eyebrow point again, tap each point approximately 7–10 times while repeating the sequence of 8 positive phrases listed below. This process enables the client to focus on solutions, with opportunity to verbalise preferences, choices, and creative outcomes. It is helpful to complete each sequence with a slow deep breath to help shift energy throughout the body.

Although tapping is the preferred method, other alternatives are required in a small percentage of cases. Feinstein et al. (2005) highlight the usefulness of massaging the points gently. Another method is called touch and breathe, which involves touching the tapping point lightly with one or two fingers and encourages the client to take a complete breath (one gentle inhalation and one gentle exhalation, usually through the nose). Then move on to the next point, synchronising the massage intervention with the client breathing freely throughout the sequence. Crucially, the client should be attuned to the factors that have been triggering the disruption in the energy system as they work through the tapping points. According to Feinstein et al. (2005: 47), 'the energy intervention is only able to rewire the unwanted feeling while it is active'. Tapping protocols can be adapted to treating a food addiction and transforming contradictory core beliefs that are prevailing (Feinstein et al. 2005).

Before I leave this section, it is worth mentioning that PSYCH-K (Williams 2004) is another interesting energy psychological technique for changing health beliefs. This is raised as a guide to health practitioners who may wish to explore William's work for comprehensive discussion including an outline of techniques.

Hit the Web for health information

In the context of changing health behaviour, the Web might be a useful source. The rapid growth in web-based healthcare information has generated numerous sites focusing on 'health lifestyle' issues. Some include interactive features, physical activity advice, personalised progress charts, e-mail access to expert advice and local community activity. The implication of this expanding universe is generally viewed as positive in regard to health promotion (Korp 2006). Interestingly, Chin

(2000) perceives the internet as another facet of the paradigm shift in healthcare. Bernhardt and Hubbey (2001) appear to recognise the vastness of information technology as revolutionary. Nonetheless, the onerous challenge for health professionals is the credibility and trustworthiness of the information given at different websites.

The notion of quality assessment and quality grading is crucial, empowering online health users to elicit reliable information. Korp (2006) notes that many health sites have significant shortcomings, as the utilisation of scientifically based criteria to assess them would be difficult. He goes on to suggest that the quality of health information is associated with the trust people place in it. Of course scientific standards of quality and trust are two distinct issues. Essentially, health professionals should attempt to construct a benchmark for good quality health information, empowering clients to make a distinction between useful and poor health information. User involvement including the expert patient could be inspirational in the identification of 'gold standard' websites. Expert patients appear to have the capacity to manage their own illness and conditions by developing knowledge relevant to maintaining health (Shaw and Baker 2004).

With fairly recent developments in 'expert patient' programmes pivotal to government plans to modernise the health service, the internet is perceived as a useful resource (DH 2001). User-led self-management programmes include challenging arthritis, self-management in asthma, and living with HIV/AIDS, and can provide important benefits for participants. Expert patient programmes are often linked with National Service Frameworks (NSF), typically coronary heart disease and long-term conditions. These programmes can help individuals to build self-efficacy and a sense of control over their daily life.

Effective management of arthritis can greatly reduce pain and disability, increase self-efficacy and improve quality of life. The conduct of focus group work with Asian women (English not being the first language) undergoing treatment for rheumatology conditions has been vividly described by Firth et al. (2005: 112–13). They revealed that the women reported difficulty accessing and understanding information regarding their condition and treatment intervention because of the language barrier. The implication is that the most truly effective health professionals will be those who recognise the needs of the ethnic minority community in the development of website material.

Expert patients looking for specific types of information will perhaps use the net in a systematic way. Some glimpses of the way the internet has been utilised by older adults with arthritis for health information can be gained from studies. A survey undertaken by Tak and Hong (2005) included 17 men and 64 women, aged 60 years and above, and pointed to interesting variables. The findings revealed that 39% sought arthritis health information on the net. Contrastingly, 61% had not used the computer to find health related information. Sending and receiving e-mails was a major activity involving 33% of the sample. Another 33% accessed the net for financial related information. The major significant factor relating to internet use was years of education (p < .009). Participants who were well educated were more likely to use the internet.

Here they found that age and functional disability resulting from arthritis did not impede internet use. Although the internet is a powerful medium for disseminating health information, Tak and Hong (2005: 137) suggest that health professionals need to refer clients to well-developed, user friendly health resources, giving consideration to readability, navigation features, credibility, organisation and graphic appearance. Also visual magnification screens and touch screens may assist people with visual impairment; a trackball or a keyboard guard is available to help with hand and finger impairments.

Health professionals need to step back and consider carefully what they can contribute to the website revolution, particularly in relation to reducing health inequalities and changing health behaviour. Although valuable websites on physical activity intervention do exist, poor participant adherence and engagement has been recognised (Leslie et al. 2005). This could be related to the capacity of service users to undertake computational tasks and utilise health related information. These issues are sturdily socially graded and seem to predict self-management in chronic disease (Mirowsky and Ross 2003). The preferences of some potential web users have been explored by Ferney and Marshall (2006) and focus on physical activity interventions. The findings are enthusiastic, emphasising the significance of design, such as constructing a home page that is easily accessible. Interactivity emerged as a crucial theme too.

A primary concern was the need for creativity to maximise user engagement, for instance, a self report progress chart allowing users to set goals and monitor physical activity progress. Another major theme alluded to providing databases on physical activity or information on specific community opportunities in local areas such as Tai Chi or walks, thus highlighting the importance of interdependence and social support as a vital ingredient in changing health behaviour. Overall, the findings of this study point to useful factors that might be helpful in the construction of a dynamic and creative website for physical activity.

Moreover, if a physical activity website is being designed to help service users with obesity problems and body image issues, additional

---

Box 9.1 Losing weight tapping sequence

Repeat one phrase for each of the tapping points (demonstrated in this box).

1. (Eyebrow) I completely appreciate feeling thin and fit.
2. (Side of eye) I could feel thin, fit and healthy.
3. (Under eye) I'm allowed to feel thin and appreciate my body.
4. (Under nose) I want to feel thin, fit and vibrant .
5. (Chin) I choose to feel thin and satisfied with my appearance.
6. (Collarbone) I allow myself to feel slender and sexy.
7. (Underarm) I allow myself to feel good about my body.
8. (Head) I appreciate my body right now.

Source: Adapted from Look (2005).

---

features should be contemplated. For example, the inclusion of nutrition might be useful, with the creation of recipes for a wide audience including vegetarians and vegans and other specific cultural preferences. Motivation readiness for changing behaviour might also be linked with the capacity for clients to manage sweet cravings and addictions. In some instances addictions are often acts of self-violation and reduce personal power to change and grow. Energy medicine techniques might be helpful to individuals attempting to overcome addictions and reach for a better sense of well-being. Clients can be encouraged to use EFT (emotional freedom techniques, www.emofree. com) and energy psychology tools (Feinstein and Eden 2005, www. innersource.net). This contemporary approach can help overcome a range of psychological problems. See Box 9.1.

Emotional well-being and intention of the health professional

It is vital, then, that health practitioners make serious attempts to engage with the psychological agenda of changing health beliefs. Despite the enormous range of literature on interpersonal and counselling skills the centrality of the health professional's emotional well-being and intention is frequently downplayed. Self-awareness is a fundamental prerequisite for facilitating dynamic interpersonal interventions. For centuries philosophers and theologians have deconstructed the meaning of 'self' with a high degree of controversy.

Existential philosophers in particular talk about 'self' from an 'ontological' position: the way of being. Sartre (1956) points to the notion of authenticity as a true and honest presentation of self in accordance with own values, feelings and desires. To be an authentic person is to live in a world where the 'being' of others is recognised and understood too. Thus in a health care context it is vital that health professionals have interactive competencies that are in touch with the patients' feelings, values and thought processes. The more challenging the resistance to changing health behaviour, the greater the need for flexible, highly responsive and empowering interactions. Crucially, the health professional's emotional state and intention are immensely important.

Scripts and emotional care

Health professionals can facilitate dysfunctional interaction with some having hidden motives for becoming involved in care work. One of the most enlightening ways of exploring the issues is through the idea of 'script', particularly as revealed by the concept of transactional analysis (Stewart and Joines 1987). The concept is a metaphor derived from the theatre, implying that the individual might be living in a way that displays similar characteristics of an actor. When in script, a professional's choices are made from a limited range, with hidden constraints on action and patterns emerging that are not consciously recognised.

Typically the rescuer caring script is commonest, attracting needy and dependent people, and perhaps the rescuer (R) is continually drawn into involvement with victim type scripts. There is a danger that this type of dysfunctional relationship can perhaps hook in a third 'player', for example, a persecutor (P) – a common enemy to unite against. The purpose of 'distance regulation' is perhaps to avoid threatening issues. There are no winners in this drama triangle (Figure 9.2). Everyone loses and feels like a victim. Stepping out of a scripted way of relating could cause extreme anxiety or feel unnatural, triggering corresponding feelings of anger or disappointment in clients because their expectations would be violated. The breakthrough might require a 'coming to consciousness' and letting go of overadaptation associated with childhood experiences and the development of a more generous attitude towards the self.

This is not simply a matter of exploring cognitive thoughts and role demands; it is also a question of feeling states and the potential to be in touch with higher vibrations. Emotional states arise mainly from thought processes. Negative thinking frequently triggers negative

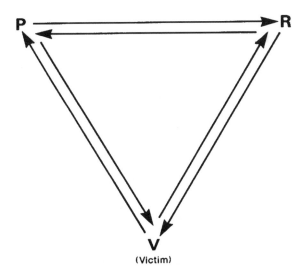

Figure 9.2 The drama triangle. Source: Karpman (1968).

emotions and a low vibrational threshold, which will affect energy flows. This could be triggered by a heavy workload, role strain, organisational change or depressive tendencies as a result of lack of love or abuse. Here, interaction between health professional and client is liable to breakdown or be unwittingly ineffective.

Contrastingly, positive thinking and high vibrational frequency will initiate and sustain positive interactions once in progress. If your subjective world is in chaos or despair or perhaps fragments of 'self' are repressed, denied or displaced, it is vital to attain a more stable equilibrium. A helpful yardstick to enable a health professional to get in touch with feeling states and develop the capacity for positive well-being is put forward by Edwards (2007). She provides an emotional scale demonstrating where emotions fall in terms of their vibrational frequency, summarised in Box 9.2.

The emotions demonstrated on this scale are indicators of a person's vibrational frequency. The higher levels display greater coherence, in tune with energy-consciousness, unleashing the power of positive intention and purpose. This is a vital ingredient if practitioners are intent on helping patients change health beliefs and improve quality of life. Contrastingly, if a health professional's vibrational frequency matches the lower end of the scale, this might represent being stuck, inner conflict or greater resistance to well-being. The mid range of the scale may be indicative of unleashing potential, shifting out of a guilt

---

Box 9.2 The emotional scale

1. Enthusiasm, freedom, empowerment, appreciation, gratitude, joy, passion, optimism, trust, intuitive knowing.
2. Calmness, acceptance, contentment, forgiveness, inner peace, patience, hopefulness, compassion.
3. Pessimism, boredom, frustration, irritation, impatience.
4. Feeling overwhelmed, busyness, worry, concern, and disappointment.
5. Self-righteousness, judgement, blame, stoicism, arrogance, anger, hatred, jealously, obsessiveness, need to control.
6. Unworthiness, guilt, insecurity, self-sacrifice, martyrdom, loneliness, feeling trapped or controlled.
7. Depression, grief, despair, fear, disempowerment.

Source: Adapted from Edwards (2007).

---

ridden, depressed or a despairing state of mind. Nonetheless, most health professionals will cycle back and forth whilst attempting to reach the higher echelons of freedom, enthusiasm, clarity and creative intention.

Deliberate intent

The notion of deliberate intent and concentrated attention is hugely significant too for health professionals who are attempting to help patients change health beliefs and promote well-being. Many health professionals often experience a heightened cognitive state but reach a threshold where the inner chatter ceases and they have a sense of focusing attentively on the client. According to McTaggart (2007) the prevailing view for manifesting intention is a heightened 'alpha' brain state. Meditation is a very helpful technique for slowing down the brain activity.

Research evidence exploring the electrical activity of the brain during meditation demonstrates a predominance of alpha rhythms (slow, high-amplitude brain waves with frequencies of 8–13 hertz), or cycles per second, which occur during light dreaming. Moreover, the theta waves slow down to 4–7 hertz, which resonates with the state of consciousness during sleep. The brain operates much faster during waking consciousness, employing beta waves, usually around 13–40 hertz.

Meditation exercises help strengthen the structure of the psyche, primarily through the cultivation of stillness and sereneness. This development enables a person to be present in the 'here-and–now', to gain poise, mindfulness, awareness and flexibility, transcending inner talk.

It is clear, then, that presenting information and facilitating education about changing health behaviour such as taking prescribed exercise requires deliberate intent from healthcare professionals. Some of the qualities and communication skills take the form of special interactive competencies. The collaborative involvement of the health professional and patient is essential, both working together, enabling the patient to reach 'concordance' in the planning and implementation of treatments (Myers and Abraham 2005). Essentially, a series of high quality interactions taking place in a context of a secure relationship is vital to help patients avoid health-risk behaviours such as smoking or unhealthy eating or explore specific beliefs and cognitions associated with changing health related behaviour. Myers and Abraham (2005) forefront a range of useful tactics for changing health behaviour and encouraging adherence to new treatment regimes. However, their exploration of this topic offers many examples related to medication, which might score virtually zero by practitioners with a mindset associated with energy psychology techniques for changing health behaviour.

Conclusions

- The challenges experienced by health professionals in attempting to change clients' health behaviour focused on shifting health beliefs, the utilisation of innovative interventions, the employment of evidenced-based practice and the intention of the practitioner.
- It is possible for health professionals with the capacity to appraise research with sufficient rigour to ascertain what is really important evidence in terms of changing health behaviour.
- The growing field of public health psychology is also a powerful source to a practitioner tackling the obesity epidemic and or smoking addictions.
- Innovative strategies for changing health beliefs have focused predominately on interventions such the potential of EFT for facilitating change.
- Emotional freedom techniques are potentially useful for breaking through addictions or changing health behaviour and promoting well-being.

- It might be useful to strengthen the provision of creative interventions in curriculum design for health professionals. Given the obesity epidemic that prevails globally and the impact of globalisation, health practitioners require insight into new conceptualisations to tackle obesity, smoking addictions and health related behaviour.
- Changing health behaviour challenges practitioners in diverse ways and offers them different opportunities for employing positive intent and reflecting on practice.
- Flexibility in the employment of different sources can be seen as a core feature of facilitating exciting behaviour change and patient empowerment. In turn, dynamic daily interventions by health practitioners have the potential to transform and determine the specific directions that change processes may take.

Further reading

Lipton B. (2005) *The Biology of Belief*. Santa Rosa, CA: Cygnus Books.
PSYCH-K website. www.psych-k.com (accessed 8 march 2008).
Williams R.M. (2004) *Psych-K. The Missing Peace in your Life*, 2nd edn. Crestone, Colo: Myrddin Books.

References

Adams J. (2007) *Researching Complementary and Alternative Medicine.* Abingdon, Oxon: Routledge.
Adams J. and Tovey P. (2008) Complementary and Alternative Medicine in Nursing Midwifery: towards a critical social science. Abingdon, Oxon: Routledge.
Arenson G. (2001) *Five Simple Steps to Emotional Healing: the last self-help book you will ever need.* New York: Fireside.
Berkman L.F., Blumenthal J., Burg M. et al. (2003) Effects of treating depression and low perceived social support on clinical events after myocardial infarction: the Enhancing Recovery in Coronary Heart Disease Patients (ENRICHD) Randomised Trial. *Journal of the American Medical Association* 289: 3106–16.
Bernhardt J.M. and Hubbey J. (2001) Health education and the Internet: the beginning of a revolution. *Health Education Research* 16: 643–5.
Bryer D.J. (2006) Influences that drive clinical decision making among junior rheumatology nurses: a qualitative study. *Musculoskeletal Care* 4(4): 223–32.
Callahan R. (2001) *Tapping the Healer Within*. London: Piatkus.
Chin R. (2000) The Internet: another facet to the paradigm shift in healthcare. *Singapore Medical Journal* 41: 426–9.

Conner M. and Norman P. (2005) *Predicting Health Behaviour*, 2nd edn. Maidenhead: Open University Press. Maidenhead.

Department of Health (DH) (2001) *The Expert Patient: A new approach to chronic disease management for the 21st century*. London: Department of Health.

Eden D. (2007) *Energy Medicine*. New York: Tarcher/Putman.

Edwards G. (2007) *Life is a Gift*. London: Piatkus.

Evans D. (2003) Hierarchy of evidence: a framework for ranking evidence evaluating healthcare intervention. *Journal of Clinical Nursing* 12(77): 84.

Feinstein D. (2005) *The Healing Power of EFT and Energy Psychology*. London: Piatkus.

Feinstein D. and Eden D. (2005) *Energy Psychology Tools*. www.innersource. net (accessed 18 February 2008).

Feinstein D., Eden D. and Craig G. (2005) The Healing Power of EFT and Energy Psychology. London: Piatkus.

Ferney S.L. and Marshall A.L. (2006) Website physical activity interventions: preferences of potential users. *Health Education Research* 21(4): 560–6.

Firth J., Newton R. and Answar S. (2005) Patients as teachers: a new approach to patient involvement. *Musculoskeletal Care* 3(2): 109–16.

Gerber R. (2001) *Vibrational Medicine*. Rochester, VA: Bear and Co.

Grypdonck M. (2006) Qualitative health research in the era of evidenced based practice. *Qualitative Health Research* 16(10): 1371–85.

Jarry J.L. and Kossert A.L. (2007) Self-esteem threat combined with exposure to thin media images leads to body image compensatory self-enhancement. *Body Image* 4: 39–50.

Karpman S. (1968) Fairy tales and script drama analysis. *Transactional Analysis Bulletin* 7(26): 39–43.

Kerr J., Weitkunat R. and Moretti M. (2005) ABC of Behaviour Change. A guide to successful disease prevention and health promotion. London: Elsevier, Churchill Livingstone.

Korp P. (2006) Health on the Internet: implications for health promotion. *Health Education Research* 21(1): 78–86.

Leslie E., Marshall A.L., Owen N. et al. (2005) Engagement and retention of participants in a physical activity website. Preventative Medicine 40: 54–9.

Lipton B. (2005) *The Biology of Belief*. Santa Rosa, CA: Cygnus Books.

Look C. (2005) *Attracting Abundance with EFT*. Blomington, Ind: Author House.

McTaggart L. (2007) *The Intention Experiment*. London: Harper Element.

Mirowsky J. and Ross C.E. (2003) *Education, Social Status and Health*. New York: Aldine De Gruyter.

Myers L. and Abraham C. (2005) Beyond 'doctor's orders'. *The Psychologist* 18(11): 680–3.

O'Becker R. (1985) *The Electric*. Georgia: Morrow.

Ring N., Coull A., Howe C., Murphy-Black T. and Watterson A. (2006) Analysis of the impact of a national initiative to promote evidence-based nursing practice. *International Journal of Nursing Practice* 12(4): 232–40.

Sartre J.P. (1956) *Being and Nothingness*. New York: Philosophical Library.

Shaw J. and Baker M. (2004) Expert patient: dream or nightmare? *British Medical Journal* 328: 723–4.

Sheldon T.A., Cullum N., Dawson D., Lankshear A., Lawson K., Watt I., West P., Wright D. and Wright J. (2004) What's the evidence that NICE guidelines have been implemented? Results from a national evaluation using time series analysis, audit of patients' notes, and interviews. *British Medical Journal* 329(7473): 999.

Steptoe A. (2004) Physical activity and mood. In N.B. Anderson (ed.) *The Encyclopedia of Health and Behaviour*. Thousand Oaks: Sage.

Stewart I. and Joines V. (1987) *TA Today. A New Introduction to Transactional Analysis*. Nottingham: Lifespace Publishing.

Tak S.H. and Hong S.H. (2005) Use of the internet for health information by older adults with arthritis. *Orthopaedic Nursing* 24(2): 134–8.

Thompson C. (2003) Clinical experience as evidence in evidence-based practice. *Journal of Advanced Nursing* 43(3): 230–7.

Thompson C. and Dowding D. (2002) Clinical Decision Making and Judgement in Nursing. Edinburgh: Churchill Livingstone.

Thompson C., Cullum N., McCaughton D., Sheldon T. and Raynor P. (2004) Nurses, information use, and clinical decision making – the real world potential for evidence-based decision in nursing. *Evidence-Based Nursing* 7: 68–72.

Upton D. and Upton P. (2005) Nurses' attitudes to evidence-based practice: impact of a national policy. *British Journal of Nursing* 14(5): 284–8.

Wardle J. and Steptoe A. (2005) *Public Health Psychology* 18(11): 672–5.

Williams R.M. (2004) PSYCK-K. Crestone, Colo: Myrddin Publications.

Index